5-28-76

c-28-76

THE HOMEMAKER'S GUIDE TO
HOME NURSING

THE HOMEMAKER'S GUIDE TO
HOME NURSING

Alice M. Schmidt, R. N.

Brigham Young University Press
Provo, Utah

Library of Congress Cataloging in Publication Data

Schmidt, Alice M   1925-
    The homemaker's guide to home nursing.

    Bibliography: p. 155
    Includes index.
    1. Home nursing.   I.   Title   [DNLM: 1.   Home
nursing.   WY195 S349h]
RT61.S28   649.8   75-34300
ISBN 0-8425-0800-7 pbk.

Library of Congress Catalog Card Number: 75-34300
International Standard Book Number: 0-8425-0800-7 (paperback)
Brigham Young University Press, Provo, Utah 84602
Second printing 1976
Printed in the United States of America
76 5Mp 19954

CONTENTS

INTRODUCTION

Having spent eight years teaching family health and home nursing at the college level, I have become increasingly aware of the inadequacy women of all ages feel toward dealing with illness in the home. They are fascinated by a class in which they can learn the basic skills necessary to care for family members. Class members who are older often comment, "Oh, I wish I had known that."

Because it is impossible for all women to avail themselves of home nursing classes, this book is an attempt to provide a ready reference for homemakers who seek answers in dealing with illness, accidents, and disaster emergencies. Some of the book was written originally as lesson material for the LDS Relief Society. All of it has been used in the college home nursing classes I teach.

Today we have many new developments, medications, and health personnel available to help us in our quest for health, but at the same time we have more people living longer as well as more people who must learn to live with chronic ailments such as diabetes and heart disease. These provide a constant challenge to the homemaker.

Since illness is no respecter of persons, all families need to learn to deal with symptoms of disease, unexpected emergencies, and simple nursing procedures. The term *home nurse* is used to refer to any family member who is giving nursing care in the home; usually it is the mother, but occasionally it is the husband, the daughter, the grandmother, or even the son. The home nurse is expected to know how to bring comfort, alleviate pain, and help the sick regain health. She should be confident and sensitive, for sick people are quite perceptive and quickly recognize and respect skilled care. A skilled home nurse is one more member of the health team who can work with doctors, nurses, and other health personnel.

There are many reasons for caring for illness in the home. With the spiraling cost of hospitalization, for example, home care is much less expensive. Also, the patient is often happier and responds more readily in a familiar environment. Or sometimes a shortage of hospital beds makes home care for less serious illnesses a necessity. And in some areas of the country hospitals and doctors are widely scattered and not readily available to everyone. The home nurse needs to know how to deal with minor accidents, how to recognize signs of illness, and how to give simple nursing care.

Several years ago I spent a few days with a friend, a semi-invalid, who was cared for by her family. Knowing that I was a nurse, they asked me to help while I was there. As I prepared to leave, my friend begged me to stay because "you know just how to help me in and out of bed." In a few minutes I was able to teach the necessary skills to other family members so that they could assist her more easily.

In addition to covering home nursing skills this book also deals with first aid, the process of aging, care of ill children, preventing illness, facing terminal illness with family members, and disaster preparation. An extended table of contents as well as an extensive index have been included to make it easier for the home nurse to locate the necessary information. Greater depth in home nursing and first aid can be obtained through taking classes offered by the American Red Cross.

By learning basic principles, using our own ingenuity, and following the guidance of available health personnel, all of us can become more skilled in assisting family members to gain and retain optimal health. Many years ago a wise man said that good health and good sense are two of life's greatest blessings. Surely the passage of time has left undimmed the wisdom of this statement; and our greatest desire as homemakers should be to help all our family members attain both good health and good sense.

PREVENTING ILLNESS

GOOD HEALTH HABITS

The World Health Organization defines health in the following way: "Health is a state of complete physical, mental and social well-being and not merely the absence of disease or infirmity." Notice that this definition helps us to understand there are many forms of illness—physical, psychological and social—which we must seek to avoid. Below are ten health habits that can help family members enjoy good health in all the areas listed in the World Health definition.

Good Posture

This health habit allows body organs to function properly and eliminates many minor aches and pains. It also leads to a better self-image and allows for higher self-esteem.

Adequate Rest

Adequate amounts of rest vary from individual to individual; each must determine for himself the right amount. Some people need only minimal amounts of sleep; others can become rested with frequent catnaps, while others require seven to eight hours daily or they become tired and grouchy. Illness, pregnancy, and other factors may increase the need for rest temporarily.

Adequate Exercise and Relaxation

Relaxation helps to restore mental equilibrium and provides social interaction. Most people find it vitally important, though as with rest, the need for relaxation may vary from person to person.

We also need sufficient exercise to allow our bodies to function optimally. How this exercise is obtained may vary considerably. Some people may get adequate exercise in their occupations—if they happen to be P.E. teachers or golf pros—but most of us must make the effort to establish an exercise program that will be implemented throughout our lives. This program should include some aerobic exercise, which improves cardiovascular-pulmonary functioning by forcing the heart and lungs to become more efficient. Aerobics such as running, cycling, walking, swimming, dancing, tennis, and rope-jumping demand large amounts of energy; and when they are done for a sustained period, they increase the capacity of the heart and lungs to function more effectively. The overall result is that the pulse rate drops and the blood vessels are more elastic. Such a program is helpful in decreasing the incidence of heart attacks and similar circulatory problems.

If you are interested in developing a personal aerobic exercise program remember these rules:

- Have a complete physical examination before embarking on a strenuous physical exercise program.
- Wear good shoes if your program involves running or jumping.
- Increase the amount of exercise gradually each week.
- Be consistent. The most effective exercise program includes exercising four or five times a week.
- Make it a lifetime effort.

More information is available in Dr. Kenneth Cooper's books on aerobics, obtainable at most bookstores in paperback form. Some university physical education departments offer courses in physical fitness that will teach you how to assess your physical condition and how to set up your own program.

Regular Medical and Dental Checkups

Every family should have a physician.

- If you are new in a community, check out the available health agencies before an emergency strikes.
- Large public libraries have a book containing the names of all medical doctors and their professional qualifications.
- Your former doctor may know the names of some of the doctors in the new community to which you are moving.
- In some communities, public health or nurse practitioner clinics are available for immunizations, physical examinations, or minor health problems.
- A family practitioner can handle most health problems.
- All family members should be encouraged to maintain adequate immunizations against communicable diseases in their area.
- Regular yearly physicals can do much to prevent or detect such problems as cancer, heart and lung disease, diabetes, and other chronic conditions.

Dental checkups should be part of the family routine. Many communities now have dentists who are specifically interested in preventive dentistry and are anxious to help families prevent dental problems as well as remedy them. We know that tooth decay and periodontal disease are both caused by bacteria in the mouth. Many dentists recommend thorough flossing and brushing of the teeth once a day to prevent these bacteria from organizing into colonies that can cause dental problems.

Avoiding Harmful Substances
- Avoidance of smoking can help to lessen the danger of cancer and emphysema.
- Other harmful substances containing drugs of various kinds should also be avoided.
- Tea, coffee, and colas contain harmful stimulants.
- Alcohol can cause severe problems in many areas of the body.
- Laxatives, some pain relievers, tranquilizers, or sedatives can develop in the user a dependence on them.
- It is best to use medicines only when they are necessary or when they are recommended by the doctor.

Awareness of Safety Hazards
This will be discussed on pages 105-108.

Avoidance of Excessive Noise, Improper Waste Disposal, and Air Pollution
We cannot all manage to move from the cities to the mountain tops, but we can all become conscious of the need to support government measures intended to give us cleaner air, less noise, and adequate water supplies and waste disposal. In some areas of the world polluted water and inadequate waste disposal are major causes of disease.

Personal Hygiene
Cleanliness among family members can do much to help prevent the spread of infection. Clean hands, individual drinking cups and silverware, daily bathing, clean clothing and hair—these are some of the things members of a family can do to help themselves remain healthy.

Good Mental Health

All of us need to be useful and independent, to love and to be loved, to accept what we cannot change. When one has good mental health he can face the world and work out solutions to his problems. Family members should be encouraged to develop a good self-image—to feel good about themselves and their relationships with other people. Good mental health includes the ability to cope with the recurrent stresses of life and to live comfortably with oneself and others in all types of situations.

Mental health is relative and varies from day to day. Sometimes poor mental health results in actual physical illness which we call psychosomatic disease (psyche, spirit, and soma, body). Doctors are learning more and more about the effect of the mind on the body and the ways in which people drain their emotions through weakened physical systems to cause illnesses such as ulcers, migraine headaches, or asthmatic attacks. Most of us have experienced psychosomatic illness in the form of weakness, nausea, or mild diarrhea when we were nervous.

Sometimes we are aware of a person who has a morbid anxiety about his health and is constantly plagued by imaginary disorders so that he goes from doctor to doctor seeking help. Such a person is called a hypochondriac. In another chapter we will discuss good mental health as it applies to the person with chronic illness.

Good Nutrition

We are what we eat, and adequate diet is extremely important if we are to remain healthy. The United States Department of Agriculture has attempted to simplify good nutrition so that the housewife need learn only about the basic four food groups. By making the appropriate selections from these food groups, she can plan adequate daily menus that will supply the necessary daily nutrients. Only a brief summary of this material is included here. If you are interested in more material on good nutrition, check with the county extension agent near you or with the U. S. Department of Agriculture.

Milk Group

Children   3 to 4 cups
Teen-agers   4 or more cups
Adults   2 or more cups

Vegetable-Fruit Group

4 or more servings include—
A citrus fruit, other fruit or
    vegetable important for
    vitamin C
A dark-green or deep-yellow
    vegetable for vitamin A —
    at least every other day
Other vegetables and fruits,
    including potatoes

Meat Group

2 or more servings
Beef, veal, pork, lamb,
    poultry, fish, eggs
As alternates — dry beans,
    dry peas, nuts

Bread-Cereal Group

4 or more servings

Whole grain, enriched,
    or restored

FAMILY HEALTH RECORDS

In addition to good health habits, each family should establish some way of keeping track of important health information about each member. Most families start a baby book for each child and include the information about medical care asked for in the book. However, since the baby book usually includes only up to age five or six, records beyond that point diminish rapidly. Thus a child in junior high school usually has to rely on less than perfect memories.

Family health records can be simple or complex and can be kept in notebooks, on cards, or in an extension to the baby book. Some doctors have booklets available in their offices that can be used. Ideally each family member would have a separate health record to take with him when necessary.

PERSONAL MEDICAL RECORD

Name _____

Birthdate _____

Family Health History:

Name	Relationship to you	Disease	Birthdate	Comment

Immunization Record

Immunization	Yr. completed	Boosters - year
DPT or TD		
Polio		
Rubeola (measles)		
Rubella (German measles)		
Mumps		
Others		

Individual Problems or Allergies

Condition	Medications	Comments

PERSONAL MEDICAL RECORD (Cont'd.)

communicable diseases, physical examinations, illnesses,
operations, dental work, x-rays

Date	Nature of illness injury, or surgery	Doctor	Office or hospital	Comments

Miscellaneous
pregnancies, blood type, RH vaccine

Date	Medical Information	Comments

Resistance and Immunity to Disease

Disease	Age at First Dose	Material (Antigen) and Dosage	Booster Doses	Adult Immunization
Diphtheria		Children 2 mos. to 6 yrs.: 3 doses at 4-6 week intervals, 4th dose approximately 1 year after third injection (DPT). School children and adults: 3 doses of TD (adult) with second dose 4-6 weeks after first and third dose 6 mos. to 1 yr. after second	Children 3 through 6 yrs.: one injection DPT intramuscularly. All other persons: TD (adult) every 10 years. If dose administered sooner as part of wound management, next booster shot not needed for another 10 yrs.	TD (adult) every 10 years: if administered sooner as part of wound management, next booster shot not needed for another 10 yrs.
Tetanus	2 months through 6 yrs.			
Whooping Cough (Pertussis)				Whooping cough not indicated after 6th year
Poliomyelitis	2 months	Sabin Oral Polio Vaccine Types 1, 111, and 11 in that order; or trivalent oral vaccine 3 doses, at 6- to 8- week intervals.	1 dose of trivalent oral vaccine at 12 to 15 months, and 1 dose on entering school.	Adults subject to unusual risk, military service, or foreign travel should receive two doses of trivalent oral vaccine 6 to 8 weeks apart.
German Measles (Rubella)	All children between age of 1 yr. and puberty. Desirable for unimmunized adolescent girls and adult women.	Live rubella virus vaccine—one dose	Probably not needed	Inadvisable or dangerous during— Pregnancy Altered immune states Severe fever Hypersensitivity: allergy to the vaccine.
Mumps	12 months of age or older.	Live mumps virus vaccine—one dose.	Probably not needed	Adolescent and adult males who have not had

8

Smallpox		Routine vaccination in unexposed populations no longer recommended since September, 1971.		Routine immunization of health personnel, travelers to and from areas where smallpox still exists.
Measles (Rubeola)	12 mo. of age or older (6 mo. in epidemic exposure)	Live attenuated measles vaccine, single dose, or live attenuated measles vaccine plus measles Immune globulin (MIG), one dose each.	Probably not needed for children vaccinated at 10-12 mo. of age or older.	Vaccination of adult rarely necessary. Precautions: Severe febrile illness Active tuberculosis Marked hypersensitivity to vaccine components Inadvisable or dangerous during altered immune states, pregnancy.
Typhoid Fever	Only when needed; routine immunization not indicated in USA.	Typhoid vaccine 2 injections 4 or more weeks apart or according to manufacturer's recommendations.	At 4-year intervals a single injection up to 2 boosters.	Only when needed; typhoid vaccine, 2 injections with single boosters at 4-year intervals: only for persons subject to risk or foreign travel.
Influenza	Annual vaccination for persons with chronic debilitating conditions.	Primary Series: 2 doses administered subcutaneously preferably 6 to 8 weeks apart, to be completed by mid-November.	Single subcutaneous dose of bivalent vaccine before mid-November for previously immunized people.	Precaution: Not administered to persons clearly hypersensitive to ingested or injected egg protein, or those who exhibit signs of a cold; may be given as the symptoms subside

(See American Medical Association Chart on Immunizations.)

Communicable Diseases

Diseases	What to look for:	Treatment	How to prevent:
Chicken Pox Incubation 14-21 days Virus	Small pimples which develop scabs by the 5th day. New pox continue to appear for several days. No longer contagious when all scabs are dry.	None. Itching may be relieved by a starch bath (1 to 2 cups of starch in a tub of water).	Prevent exposure. No immunization available.
Diphtheria Incubation 2 to 5 days	Sore throat, patches on tonsils and throat.	Medical treatment and supervision.	Immunization during infancy.
German Measles (Rubella) Incubation 14-21 days Virus	Rash on face and hands spreading to the body and lasting 2 to 3 days. Glands at back of head along the neck are enlarged. Slight fever.	Keep child comfortable	Gamma globulin is used to give temporary protection to unprotected pregnant women. Available permanent immunization.
Impetigo Staphylococcus infection of the skin.	Thick oozing scabs or crusts, usually on the face.	Antibiotic cream prescribed by a doctor. Child should be isolated and prevented from scratching.	Prevent exposure to children having impetigo.
Infectious Hepatitis Variable incubation Virus	Weakness, fever, headache, nausea, vomiting followed by jaundice.	Bed rest, medical supervision.	Prevent contact with previous cases. Polluted water or food may cause infection. Gamma globulin will give temporary protection.
Measles (Rubeola) Incubation 9 to 12 days Virus	High fever, cold symptoms, inflamed eyes. Rash appears in 3 to 4 days.	Bed rest, adequate fluids. Watch for serious complications.	Prevent contact. Use gamma globulin following exposure. Permanent immunity available.
Meningitis Incubation 2 to 10 days Bacteria	Vomiting, headache, stiff neck. Fever.	Prompt medical attention.	Prevent exposure.

Disease / Incubation	Symptoms	Treatment	Prevention
Mumps Incubation 14 to 28 days Virus	Fever, swelling of parotid glands at the angle of the jaw.	Bed rest during acute phase. Check with doctor to determine diagnosis.	Permanent immunity available.
Pinkeye (Conjunctivitis) Bacteria	Red eyes and purulent discharge. Eyelids may be stuck together in the morning.	Antibiotic drops or ointment prescribed by doctor.	Highly contagious. Good personal hygeine—separate towels.
Pinworms	Itching in the area surrounding the anus, particularly at night. Child cries and is very restless about 1 to 2 hours after going to sleep. Worms appear as tiny, short threads near the anal sphincter.	Notify doctor to obtain medication. Clean underclothing daily. Change bed linens regularly.	Teach children to wash their hands before eating and after using the toilet.
Ringworm of the scalp Incubation 10 to 14 days Fungus	Circular patches of rough skin about the size of a nickel. Hair is broken off short in the center of the infection.	Medical treatment is necessary.	Avoid using infected combs or exchanging hats or caps.
Salmonellosis Incubation 6 to 72 hours after eating contaminated food or water.	Acute diarrhea, nausea, and vomiting, cramping, dehydration.	Nothing by mouth during vomiting, clear liquids during diarrhea. Check with doctor if dehydration occurs.	Avoid contaminated food or water.
Scabies Incubation 4 to 8 days Mites	Itching—worse at night. Fine lines or burrows usually between fingers or toes or in the armpit.	Medical treatment prescribed and repeated in 24 hours.	Cleanliness—frequent bathing. Clean clothing and bedding.
Strep Throat Incubation 2 to 5 days Bacteria	Headache, fever, sore throat, swollen neck glands. Fine diffuse rash occurs with scarlet fever.	Antibiotics—check with the doctor.	Prevent exposure. Medical treatment of severe sore throats.
Whooping cough Incubation 5 to 8 days	Cold symptoms, long coughing spells especially at night, followed by vomiting.	Medical treatment and supervision.	Immunization during infancy.

Although each family might find that the information they wish to keep is slightly different, the following general categories are important:

- Immunizations—with appropriate booster dates
- Communicable diseases—dates and any complications
- Hospitalizations—including the date and name of hospital
- Operations—including the date, doctor's name and name of hospital
- Height and weight during the growing years
- Serious illnesses—including a brief summary of the length of the illness and any pertinent information
- Physical and dental examinations—dates
- X-rays—date, type, and where taken
- Major dental work—wisdom teeth pulled, orthodontic work
- Blood type—if known
- Allergies of all kinds—food, dust, pollen, medicines, and others

Family health records should be readily available, up-to-date, and legible.

PROTECTING FAMILY MEMBERS

No way has been found to guarantee a family complete freedom from illness, but certain rules can help avoid communicable disease.

- Whenever possible, avoid direct contact with those who are ill.
- Have separate personal items such as toothbrushes, combs, and towels for each family member. Using another person's drinking glass, eating with his fork, sharing foods such as ice cream cones or candy, and kissing are frequent methods of spreading disease.
- Teach family members to cover their noses and mouths with handkerchiefs or tissues when they sneeze or cough. Organisms travel only a few inches with breathing, but they may be expelled several feet with a vigorous sneeze or cough, contaminating all those nearby.
- Wash your hands before preparing food or eating, after going to the toilet, after helping a sick person, and after playing with pets.
- Use safe water, milk, and other foods. Keep perishable food refrigerated to prevent bacteria from multiplying. When camping, use only pure water; boil or disinfect questionable water before using.

- Maintain proper immunization.
- Watch for symptoms of illness among family members so that an infectious person can be isolated before a disease is spread. We will discuss this at greater length in chapter three.

EMERGENCY PREPAREDNESS

Each family should also prepare itself for disaster situations. A good plan is to have a supply of food and other necessary items on hand so that a family can be self-sustaining in case of famine or economic adversity. Some families stockpile only basic foods such as wheat, sugar, salt, and powdered milk, while others use a rotating supply of all their regular foods. Many booklets are available to help families determine quantities and rotation plans for such supplies. Two of these are "Family Food Stockpile for Survival," Home and Garden Bulletin No. 77, U.S. Department of Agriculture and *In Time of Emergency* by the Department of Defense.

Food and Water

The United States Civil Defense authorities encourage all families to have a two-week supply of food and water in order to be self-sufficient in the event of a natural disaster where transportation must be reestablished or an atomic disaster where radiation would keep rescuers out of the area for up to two weeks.

About one-half gallon of water per person per day is optimal for drinking. Minimal handwashing and personal hygiene could be accomplished with another half gallon per person per day. Thus a family should plan on storing fourteen gallons per person for a two-week supply. There are a number of ways to store water:

- Plastic jugs may be thoroughly cleaned, filled with water, and capped with a tight-fitting lid. Plastic containers are shatter proof and lighter than glass. Metal containers may give the water an unpleasant taste.
- Clean fruit jars may be filled with water, leaving one inch of headspace at the top of the jar. These jars should be processed in a water bath in the same way that fruit juice is processed, allowing twenty minutes for quart jars and twenty-five minutes for two-quart jars. These will remain sterile for several years but should be inspected periodically. When cloudiness, odors or objectionable flavors develop, a fresh supply should be processed. After a disaster, you will want to treat water to make it

Guide for Reserve Food Supply

Kind of food	Need per person		Remarks
	Daily	2 weeks	
1. Milk	Equivalent of 2 glasses (fluid)	Equivalent of 7 qts. (fluid)	Each of the following is about the equivalent of one quart of fluid milk: Three 6-oz. cans of evaporated milk. One 14½ oz. can of evaporated milk. Three to 3½ ozs. of nonfat dry milk.
2. Canned meat, poultry, fish dry beans, and peas	2 servings	28 servings (about 8 to 9 lbs.)	Amounts required for one serving of each food are as follows: Canned meat, poultry, fish—2 to 3 ozs. Canned mixtures of meat, poultry, or fish with vegetables, rice, macaroni, spaghetti, noodles, or dry beans—8 ozs. Thick soups containing meat, poultry, fish or dry beans or peas—one-half of a 10½-oz. can (condensed).
3. Fruits and vegetables	3 to 4 servings	42 to 56 servings (about 21 lbs. canned)	Amounts required for one serving of each food are as follows: Canned juices—4 to 6 ozs., single strength. Canned fruit and vegetables—4 ozs. Dried fruit—1½ ozs.
4. Cereals and baked goods	3 to 4 servings	42 to 56 servings (about 5 to 7 lbs.)	Amounts required for one serving of each food are as follows (selection depends on extent of cooking possible): Cereal: Ready-to-eat, puffed—½ oz. Ready-to-eat, flaked—¾ oz. Other ready-to-eat and uncooked—1 oz. Crackers, cooking—1 oz. Canned bread, steamed puddings, and cake—1 to 2 ozs. Flour, flour mixes—1 oz. Macaroni, spaghetti, noodles: Dry—¾ oz.

5.	Spreads for bread and crackers	According to family practices	Examples:
			Cheese spreads.
			Peanut and other nut butters.
			Jam, jelly, marmalade, preserves.
			Syrup, honey.
			Apple and other fruit butters.
			Relish, catsup, mustard.
6.	Hydrogenated fats and vegetable oils	Up to 1 lb. or 1 pt.	Amount needed depends upon extent of cooking possible.
7.	Sugars, candy, nuts, instant puddings	1 to 2 lbs.	
8.	Miscellaneous	According to family practices	Examples (amount needed depends on extent of cooking possible):
			Instant beverages.
			Instant, dry cream substitute.
			Bouillon products.
			Synthetic beverage products.
			Salt and spices (e.g., pepper).
			Flavoring extracts, vinegar.
			Soda, baking powder.
9.	Water (for drinking)	½ gal. 7 gals.	

safe. You may either add two or three drops of tincture of iodine to each quart of water or disinfect it with chlorine, according to the following chart.

Dosage of Chlorine Solution for Disinfecting Drinking Water

	Dosage of 5.25% sodium hypochlorite solution for—	
Gallons of water	Clear water	Cloudy water
¼ (one quart)	1 drop	3 drops
1	4 drops	10 drops
5	¼ teaspoon	½ teaspoon

In preparation for disaster

Know these things:

- Where to find safe water
- How to turn off water service valve
- How to purify water
- What foods to store and how to prepare them
- What foods are unsafe
- How to dispose of garbage
- How to dispose of human wastes
- What to do with frozen foods

Have these things:

- Stored water (14 gals. per person)
- Two-week's supply of food, paper plates, and napkins
- Cooking and eating utensils, measuring cup, can and bottle openers, pocket knife, and matches
- Baby food
- Large garbage can for garbage
- Smaller can for human wastes
- Covered pail for bathroom purposes
- Toilet tissue, paper towels, sanitary napkins, disposable diapers, soap
- Medicine and special equipment for the sick
- Grocery bags, newspapers for sanitary uses, waterproof gloves
- Two pints household chlorine
- Wrench, screwdriver, shovel and crowbar

- Candles
- Flashlight and batteries
- A battery-operated radio
- Bedding and extra clothing

For further information concerning the lists above, refer to a booklet issued by the Department of Defense: "Home Protection Exercises."

SUMMARY

Each of us wishes to be healthy in order to enjoy life more fully. By practicing good health habits, keeping good health records, and carrying out routine precautions, we may be able to achieve this goal most of the time.

TREATING ILLNESS

Every family must deal with illness at one time or another. Sometimes the patient is cared for in the hospital, but more often home care is adequate. This decision is arrived at in a conference between the family and the doctor. With the rising costs of hospitalization, the earlier mobility following surgery and childbirth, the increasing lifespan, and the growing emphasis on home care for long-term illness, family members find themselves filling the role of home nurse with increasing frequency. A home nurse is a nonprofessional person caring for illness in the home. Usually the home nurse is the wife and mother, but husbands, sons, daughters, and sometimes friends may also find themselves in this role. The next few chapters will introduce you to home-nursing skills that can be of benefit when family members are ill.

BASIC NURSING PRINCIPLES

Five basic nursing principles, if followed, will guarantee good patient care in the home:

- Safety: A home nurse is concerned about the safety of the patient, the home nurse herself, other family members, and any visitors to the home. If she uses poor body mechanics in turning the patient, she has failed to think about her own safety. If she gives wrong medication, she has failed to consider the patient's safety. Preventing the spread of disease is also a safety principle discussed later in detail.
- Comfort: Most of the care a home nurse gives involves comfort. A smooth bed, a good backrub, a change of position—these are comfort measures. The patient usually remains in the hospital during the time he needs extensive or intensive care and treatment, and when he returns home, the home nurse seeks to promote his well-being and recovery by keeping him comfortable.
- Effectiveness: If a procedure is not effective, there is no point in doing it. If you have not removed the wrinkles under the patient when tightening the sheet, the procedure is ineffective.

A thermometer which is used without first shaking it down may give an inaccurate reading. An incorrect medication is not effective and may also be unsafe. There are many ways to do any given nursing skill, and the basic test is whether the procedure is effective.

- Neatness: This principle is particularly important in the sick room since it not only facilitates cleanliness but also boosts the patient's morale. An untidy room may cause the patient to ask himself two questions: Am I too great a burden on the family? Doesn't the home nurse care about me enough to keep things neat? Either of these conclusions on the part of the patient may cause him great anxiety. Although illness may drastically disrupt family routines, the home nurse should make every effort to keep the sickroom neat.

- Economy: This principle involves more than money. It involves time, effort, and planning for household supplies. Suppose you had a bedfast patient in your home for a few weeks. Would you need to buy or rent expensive hospital equipment, or could you improvise? The last chapter in this book will be devoted to explaining ways in which equipment may be improvised. Most such equipment is not so versatile and effective as professional equipment, and the family will need to decide which will fit its situation best. When the family is dealing with long-term patient care, professional equipment may be the most economical in terms of energy expended and comfort for both the home nurse and the patient.

These nursing fundamentals are the guidelines to successful home nursing. Taken together, the first letters of the five words spell SCENE—an easy way to remember safety, comfort, effectiveness, neatness, and economy. Without all of them the home nurse finds herself doing less than her best in caring for illness among family members.

SETTING UP THE SICK ROOM

A Separate Room

If an effort is being made to protect other family members, or if the doctor has suggested bed rest for the person who is ill, a separate room should be provided for the patient. It should be a quiet, pleasant room, preferably near the bathroom. All unnecessary items should be removed from the room to facilitate cleaning and to eliminate clutter. A comfortable chair or two left in the room will encourage family members to stop and chat with the patient occasionally.

The Bed

A single-size bed will facilitate nursing care since the patient can be reached easily from either side. If the patient is confined to bed, the bed should be raised to the height of the home nurse's hips. This will allow her to care for the patient without straining her back and shoulders. Electric hospital beds allow the bed to be raised or lowered as needed. A standard single bed can be raised by several techniques:

- Adding an extra mattress
- Using wooden blocks made by the home handyman
- Making stacks of books, magazines, or newspapers to put under each leg (each stack tied securely)
- Placing under each bed leg a can or bucket filled with sand, dirt, or gravel (the lid of the can or a piece of wood placed on top of the sand to prevent the bed leg from working its way downward)

With each of the above methods, except number one, the casters should be removed to make the bed more stable.

The Mattress

The mattress should be firm and in some cases may need to be protected by a waterproof cover. A bed board made of 3/4" plywood placed between the springs and the mattress will make the surface of the bed firm and level. Bedding should be clean, soft, lightweight, and easily washable. Contoured bottom sheets stay wrinkle-free longer but will wear out more quickly.

Temperature and Light

The sickroom should be kept comfortably warm but not hot. A humidifier will make the room feel comfortable at a lower temperature. Light should not shine directly into the patient's eyes.

Bedside Items

At the bedside the patient should have tissue wipes and a waste container, a pitcher of water or juice and a glass, a bed bag for small personal items (See page 155 for construction), and recreational materials according to the age of the patient. Be sure the patient has some means of calling the home nurse since it is demeaning for the patient to have to yell for help. A small bell, two lids, a whistle, a baseball bat to bang on the floor, or a Halloween noisemaker would work satisfactorily.

PREVENTING THE SPREAD OF INFECTION

Waste Disposal

Adequate waste disposal is vitally important in preventing the spread of infection. Tissues, dressings, uneaten food, and body excreta must all be dealt with. The first three items can be handled adequately in newspaper or grocery sacks. When using a grocery sack, make a 1½- to 2-inch cuff at the top. This helps to prevent the sack from collapsing and allows the home nurse to pick up the sack under the cuff to avoid touching the contaminated top edge; and, with a small sack, it makes a convenient flap to pin to the sheet at the bedside.

Most homemakers have a stack of newspapers available from which newspaper bags can be made. These are very useful pinned to the side of the bed as a receptacle for tissues. The procedure is as follows (fig. 1):

- Fold the newspaper in half on a flat surface with the fold toward you.
- Turn the upper edge of the top half down to the fold.
- Turn the paper over, keeping the bottom fold toward you.
- Fold each side so that the paper is folded in thirds.
- Tuck one side under the cuff of the other side to lock the bag.
- Fold the top flap down. This flap can be pinned to the bed or used as a cover when disposing of the bag.

Handwashing

We mentioned in chapter one the necessity for adequate handwashing as a method of preventing illness. When illness does occur, the home nurse must take extra care in the handwashing technique. She should always wash before and after care of the patient since this will help to protect him from outside organisms and will protect the family from organisms harbored by the patient.

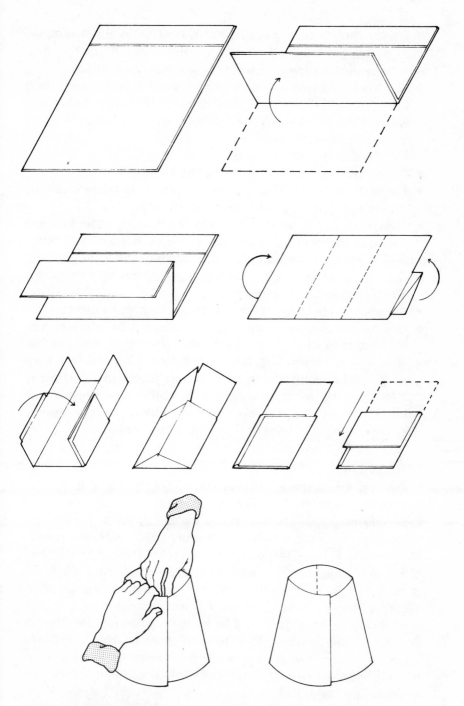

Fig. 1. Newspaper receptacle

Ideally, the home nurse should have access to running water, though handwashing may be done with water poured from a pitcher by another family member. The procedure is as follows:

- Wet the hands with lukewarm water, since water hot enough to kill bacteria (150°–180°) would burn the hands. Lukewarm water feels comfortable and makes the nurse's hands warm enough to touch the patient.
- Pick up the soap and work up a lather.
- Rinse the bar of soap before replacing it in the soap dish.
- Lather all surfaces of the hands. Remember to get between the fingers and thumbs and to include the wrists.
- Hold your hands downward under the running water to allow the soap to be rinsed away. Do not use a stopper in the sink, and do not touch the water in the bottom of the basin.
- Repeat the procedure a second time, remembering to rinse the bar of soap before placing it in the soap dish.
- Be sure to rinse away all the soap to avoid chapped hands.
- Dry the hands thoroughly. If you are using a paper towel, you may use it to turn off the water, thus preventing recontamination of the hands. Use lotion if desired. Chapped hands are rough and uncomfortable, and the tiny cracks that occur may allow bacteria to penetrate the skin. If the nurse's hands have become chapped and cracked, a spring clothespin may be used to pick up soiled tissues or dressings from a wound.

Protective Apron

Wearing a protective, coverall apron is a third way to prevent the spread of infection. This is used only when the patient is definitely isolated from the rest of the family either for his own protection (as in the case of a premature baby) or for the protection of the family. In order for the coverall apron to be most effective it should be long enough to cover the front of the home nurse's dress or shirt and should open in the back. Instead of an apron, a man's short-sleeved shirt worn backwards or a brunch coat might be used. It should be hung on a hanger near the sick room with the contaminated front part away from the traffic flow. The apron is worn only when the home nurse must come in contact with the patient or the bed. The procedure is as follows:

- Wash your hands.
- Hold the apron at the top and slip into it without touching the

contaminated front area. It should be securely fastened in the back with snaps or ties so that it will not flap around.

- After the patient has been cared for, wash your hands again before removing the apron.
- Unfasten the apron.
- Slip out of it without touching the front part.
- Place the apron back on the hanger with the opening facing outward ready for the next use.

The apron should be washed when it becomes wet or soiled and after it is no longer needed for patient care.

A DAILY RECORD

When a family member is seriously ill, under the direct care of a doctor, or being cared for by more than one person, a daily record facilitates nursing care. It should contain a chronological record of how the patient feels, and how he reacts, what care has been given, and any pertinent observations that might enhance the patient's care. (A sample daily record is shown in fig. 2.)

The doctor's orders should be written on the back of the daily record. It is best to clarify with him any orders not plainly understood by the home nurse. For example: What does the doctor mean by bed rest? Does he mean that the patient must have everything done for him (must he be bathed, shaved and fed)? Or does it mean that he can do anything as long as he stays in bed? Or does it mean that he can walk to the bathroom but must remain in bed the rest of the time?

CARING FOR THE SICK CHILD

Remember that most childhood illnesses are caused by infectious organisms and the child usually becomes ill very quickly. Most parents come to recognize how each child in the family will react to illness. Many children between six and adolescence are very upset when they become ill. They may even fear death if they are seriously ill. They need a great deal of emotional support and understanding as well as an explanation of what is happening and what the outcome will be.

Keep in mind that children live in the present, easily forget the past, and are not concerned about the future. Their attention span is very short, either for pain or pleasure. They are readily interested in sights, sounds, and food. They need especially to know

DAILY RECORD

SUSAN SMITH

DATE and HOUR	T. P. R.	DIET, MEDICINE and TREATMENT	B.M.	URINE	REMARKS
MAY 10					
8:30 PM	101.^{2} 96-24	GLASS OF ORANGE JUICE		✓	COMPLAINS OF SORE THROAT. SAYS SHE ACHES.
9:00 PM		RX 5692 1 TAB.			
12:00 M	102 98-26	ASPIRIN 2 TAB.		✓	VERY RESTLESS.
MAY 11					
5:00 AM	101.^{8} 94-24	ASPIRIN 2 TAB.	✓	✓	
8:00 AM		SOFT DIET			ATE VERY LITTLE
9:00 AM	100 88-22	ASPIRIN 2 TAB. RX 5692 1 TAB. GLASS OF LEMONADE		✓	RESTING BETTER THROAT LESS SORE
10:00 AM			✓		UP TO B.R. DIZZY. B.M. VERY RUNNY.
12:00 N	100.^{2} 90-22	LIQUID DIET		✓	TOOK WELL.
1:00 PM					SLEEPING.
4:00 PM	99.^{8} 84-20	GLASS 7-UP		✓	FEELS BETTER.

DOCTORS ORDERS

SCHEDULE

DIET AS DESIRED
UP TO BATHROOM
ASPIRIN 2 TAB. EVERY 4 HRS. AS NEEDED
RX 5692 1 TAB. TWICE DAILY   9:00 AM 9:00 PM

DR. JONES

Fig. 2. Patient's daily record

that someone cares and will help them when they need it. A sick child cannot be spoiled. Give him extra love and attention.

When a child becomes ill, observe the following guidelines:

- Keep the child as quiet as possible. A sick baby may need to be held and rocked to soothe him. Rest is important to recovery.
- Keep other family members away until the illness has been diagnosed.
- Withhold all food if the child is vomiting, but if vomiting continues more than a few hours, watch for dehydration (no urine, and a dry mouth).
- Let the child's appetite be the guide in giving him food, but be sure he gets adequate liquids.
- Check with the doctor if the diagnosis is in question, if the fever is unusually high, or if dehydration becomes evident. Usually it is better not to give medications (except aspirin) without the doctor's instructions.
- Keep a record of temperature, vomiting, bowel movements, medicine given, food and fluids taken, and any unusual observations (stiff neck, pulling on the ear, difficulty swallowing, rash).

If a child must be hospitalized, it is often a traumatic experience. It may help if a parent can be with him initially. If not, he should be told what it will be like. He should not be told there will be no pain; on the other hand, telling him everything that will be done may be unduly frightening. Convalesence is a time that particularly challenges the ingenuity of the home nurse as she seeks to keep a child happily occupied.

Diversions for Younger Children

- Mobiles or a bulletin board with a new picture every day
- A hamster or similar pet in a cage
- A sweet potato vine or carrot top growing in a glass jar
- Goldfish or tropical fish in a tank nearby
- Cutting paper dolls
- Magic slates
- Chains of paper clips, paper circles, spools, buttons, or macaroni
- Magnets or a magnifying glass
- Picture puzzles or simple games
- Clay (homemade: 1 C. flour, 1 C. salt, 1 tbsp. alum. Add 3/4 to 1 C. water which has been tinted with food coloring. Let stand in a jar overnight before using. Store in a tight container.)

Diversions for Older Children in Addition to Those Above
- A caterpillar becoming a butterfly; a tadpole
- Basketry, braiding, carving, ceramics, felt craft, hooked rugs, jewelry, leather craft, models of all kinds, pipe cleaner animals and flowers, puppets, stamp collecting, weaving, knitting
- Reading or telling stories to younger family members
- Helping plan menus
- Using a dictaphone or telephone or tape recorder

PSYCHOLOGICAL ASPECTS OF ILLNESS

When a person is physically well and emotionally healthy, his body functions smoothly, and he usually adjusts readily to his environment; but when illness strikes, anxiety occurs. Think of how you have felt when you were ill, particularly if you didn't know what was wrong or if you were faced with major surgery, loss of a body part, hospitalization, or a disease for which there is no known cure, such as terminal cancer, diabetes, or arthritis. Perhaps you felt helpless and dejected, irritable, or worried. If you have never experienced these feelings, it may be difficult for you to understand a family member in this situation.

Illness is often accompanied by unconscious and often unrealistic fears as well as threats to the patient's ego. The illness tends to occupy the victim's thoughts completely, and he may become narcissistic and withdrawn. Regression is common as the patient concentrates on his body and its needs. Even with a simple illness, a child may become apathetic, curling up in a corner and remaining quiet. Perhaps this is a necessary mechanism allowing all the body cells to concentrate on the battle with illness.

Sometimes a patient becomes angry when he is ill because of the dependency forced upon him by his physical weakness and limited mobility. He resents being bathed and dressed, pushed and pulled. Even his body elimination is no longer private as he is forced to ask for the bedpan or the urinal. Is it any wonder then that the bedfast patient is often constantly complaining or demanding as he seeks desperately to maintain his independence and enhance his ego?

Even a patient who seems outwardly cheerful may be hiding his fears and anger and may desperately need an opportunity to talk out things he has supressed. The depressed patient also bears watching. These patients can be recognized by signs such as lack of enthusiasm, prolonged insomnia, listlessness, reluctance to speak, neglect of appearance, withdrawal, lack of interest in anything, and feelings of worthlessness. He may even consider suicide as he seeks to get away from an overwhelming situation. Depression can usually be overcome by a willing listener, but if the patient talks about suicide, be sure to alert the doctor so that together you can plan an approach to prevent such a drastic action.

The family's feelings about a patient's illness are also vitally important. The patient needs love and empathy, which includes understanding and a desire to help, not just sympathy or feeling sorry. You do not have to have experienced the same illness as the patient to have empathy, but you do have to be accepting and nonjudgmental of his feelings and actions.

Consider the following guidelines in dealing with a patient:

- Be yourself. Sick people are anxious, but they are also very perceptive and suspicious. If you are genuine, they feel they can trust you. Be positive and show genuine interest.
- Small points of care are important. Nothing is too small to escape the patient's notice when he is concentrating on himself.
- Don't just talk; size up the situation. What is the patient expressing? Does he seem worried or withdrawn? What is his attitude toward you? Give the patient an opening such as "How are things going?" Reflect his responses to give him an opportunity to say more. Don't tell him how he *should* feel or you cut off the communication.
- Also, don't try to talk him out of the way he feels. Somehow we have the idea that the home nurse should be perpetually cheerful and should seek to make the patient feel that way. If he says he feels terrible, let him, but encourage him to tell you why. You do not need to be able to solve all of his problems, but you need to let him talk about them.
- Help the patient gather as many facts about his condition as possible, and help him to learn the skills necessary to live with his illness. This may mean you will have to find sources of information outside the family so that you can be a resource for the patient. We are always less frightened of things we know something about, and that is true with disease as with other conditions in life.
- If the patient asks no questions or seems reluctant to talk, do not pry. Explain what you are doing as you care for him and

give him plenty of opportunity to ask questions should he choose to do so.

- Don't use such clichés as "Don't worry," or "Everything will be all right." These worry a patient even more. Instead, give him every opportunity to express his doubts and fears. Just talking about them will make him feel better.
- Don't be too quick to give advice. Help the patient to make his own decisions and be responsible for them.
- NEVER talk down to a patient, even though he is disoriented or confused. If he is an adult, he should be treated as one.
- A patient needs to know that someone cares about him, but don't smother him with attention; and don't do things for him that he can do for himself.
- When a patient is angry, allow him to be, even though it may seem as though the anger is directed at you. Keep your senses in tune so that you know when he is bored, angry, or anxious.

Occasionally a person facing serious illness loses complete physical and emotional control because of his inability to accept what is happening to him. This may be a time when he begins to question his religious faith. It is a time when he may need to keep in close touch with his church to maintain inner peace and gain the courage to face his illness.

Isolation from friends and from normal activity is usually felt keenly during illness, especially if the illness lasts a long time. Every effort should be made to make the ill person feel part of the family. If he can be out of bed, he should be brought to the table at mealtimes or have someone take a tray and eat with the patient in his room. A mirror positioned just right may allow the patient to see into another room. Diversion is important but should not be tiring and should follow the patient's natural inclinations.

COMMUNITY HEALTH AGENCIES

Every home nurse should be aware of agencies in her community that can help her with health problems in her family. In larger communities the Red Cross may offer courses in first aid, home nursing, and parent preparation. Local health departments may have inexpensive immunization clinics, well-baby clinics, and health supervision for school children. They may also supply health literature. Most health departments have professional nurses on their staffs who are available to visit homes and instruct family members in special care of the sick.

SUMMARY

When illness does occur in the family, a family council should be called and plans made to distribute the additional responsibilities that may arise. The home nurse should organize her work to avoid tension and strain. Perhaps this will mean leaving some things undone for awhile. All family members who can help should be taught the necessary nursing skills since competence reassures the patient and makes him more comfortable.

RECOGNIZING ILLNESS

It is important that the home nurse recognize signs and symptoms indicating a change in the health status of a family member. *Signs* are objective and can be evaluated by the nurse herself. Examples include fever, rash, vomiting, change in skin color or pulse rate, and coughing or wheezing. *Symptoms,* on the other hand, are subjective and include such things as pain, nausea, malaise, aching, and listlessness. The two terms, however, are often used interchangeably so that we often say the "symptoms" of a cold include a runny nose and a fever, both of which are actually visible signs.

The home nurse must learn to be observant, to listen closely, and to ask pertinent questions in order to gather the necessary information to determine the nature and seriousness of the illness. If the illness is serious enough to require medical attention, the doctor may use laboratory techniques to help him make or confirm a diagnosis.

Since most of the illnesses occurring during childhood are caused by infectious organisms that cause a rise in temperature, a child tends to become ill rather suddenly. He may have been playing about as usual but begins to complain or seems suddenly tired or feels hot to the touch. Since very young children cannot tell us what is bothering them, observation becomes even more important. The child may pull on his ear if it hurts or may draw up his legs when he has abdominal pain.

Older people seem to be more subject to illnesses that come on gradually and may not be accompanied by fever. Examples include heart disease, emphysema, arthritis, and diabetes. In very elderly people, sensations may be diminished, or observed changes may simply be due to the aging process; so once again observation becomes vitally important.

PHYSICAL IRREGULARITIES

Skin

The skin should be observed for changes in color, and the home nurse must determine whether the change is normal or abnormal.

Redness occurs normally following a hot shower, exercise, or embarrassment. Abnormally it may indicate fever, injury, infection, or inflammation. The body's response to injury or infection includes sending increased fluid to an area, allowing additional white cells to be present to attack the infection or to take care of the damaged cells. Increased fluid in the area results in heat, swelling, redness, and pain. The home nurse should recognize this process and should seek to determine whether it is due to injury, infection, or inflammation.

Pallor (paleness of the skin) may occur when a person is frightened or tired. As a sign of illness it occurs when a patient faints, vomits, or is in shock. Pallor reflects a lack of blood to an area.

Jaundice (yellowness of the skin and whites of the eyes) is a symptom of disease, not a disease itself. Occasionally we see a slight jaundice in newborn babies which is considered normal, but in other instances jaundice usually indicates serious problems in the liver or the bile system. It is often seen with hepatitis, cirrhosis of the liver, cancer of the liver, and certain gall bladder diseases. All of these diseases should be treated by a physician.

Cyanosis means a blue tinge to the skin. It occurs when there is a lack of oxygen in the blood or a lack of circulation to an area. We see it commonly in a person who is extremely cold, in a child who has a temper tantrum, and in the legs of an elderly person who has poor circulation. People with emphysema, heart disease, or circulatory problems may become cyanotic around the lips when they overexert themselves. All babies are cyanotic when they are born but usually become pinkish-red as they begin to breathe on their own.

In addition to color changes, the skin should be observed for temperature, excessive dryness (seen in dehydration), excessive perspiration (seen during a high fever), and changes of texture (seen with eczema, psoriasis, or other forms of dermatitis).

Eyes

Are the eyes dull or bright? Are the whites of the eyes yellow?

Are they sensitive to light? Are they red and inflamed?

The eyes may be inflamed due to rubbing, allergies, the presence of a foreign body, or infection called conjunctivitis. Conjunctivitis is usually accompanied by pain and the presence of pus in the eyes. It is easily spread from one person to another if they use the same towel and washcloth. It usually responds quickly to an antibiotic ointment or drops prescribed by the doctor.

Some diseases are characterized by a disturbance of vision, and the doctor should be notified when a family member complains of blurred vision, double vision, limited vision, spots before his eyes, sensitivity to light, excessive watering, or pain.

1921595

Nose and Throat

Most of us are familiar with the symptoms of illness found in the nose and throat. The nose may be runny or stopped up and the throat may be red, swollen, spotted, and sore. Unfortunately, many communicable diseases begin with a sore throat so that it is difficult to distinguish a cold from a more serious disease. Usually a person with a sore throat should be kept separate from other family members in order to prevent the spread of disease.

Digestion

Nausea, vomiting, and abdominal cramps are familiar symptoms to most home nurses. They may indicate flu, food poisoning, appendicitis, infections, or pregnancy, and the home nurse needs to implement observation with pertinent questions. Continued weight loss in the absence of dieting may also be a sign of illness.

Body Elimination

Diarrhea, constipation, blood-tinged stools or urine, frequency of urination or burning upon urination are all unusual and should be reported to the doctor if they continue for a period of time. Two of the common signs of diabetes are excessive thirst and excessive urination.

Vital Signs

Temperature, pulse and respiration are what we call vital signs. They give us some indication of how the body is functioning. If a doctor is contacted, he usually asks the home nurse if she has taken the patient's temperature.

Pain

Pain is an important symptom of illness and should not be disregarded. However, it is subjective, and the home nurse should do some questioning as to location, type (stabbing, intermittent, throbbing, or aching, severity, time of onset, and possible causes. A child who complains of abdominal pain early in the morning may be trying to avoid school, may have done fifty sit-ups in physical education yesterday, or may be the victim of food poisoning or other illness. Abdominal pain accompanies many serious conditions. If it occurs, the home nurse should not give an enema or laxative or medication for pain until after checking with the doctor.

Remember that the aged seem less sensitive to all forms of pain and may tend to minimize it. Remember also that each family member responds differently to pain.

Behavior

Most infectious illnesses are accompanied by general discomfort, fatigue, and weakness called malaise. Some long-term illnesses such as anemia, leukemia, brain tumors, or mental illness may cause general prolonged behavioral changes such as fatigue, irritability, memory loss, or personality changes.

The ability to observe, question, and determine the severity of illness comes with practice and experience. Knowing individual family members as well as she does may make the home nurse invaluable in assisting the doctor to evaluate symptoms. Usually the doctor's diagnosis is based on a physical examination, laboratory tests, and answers to questions from the patient and family.

The Seven Danger Signals of Cancer

Some physical irregularities that should never be ignored are the seven signs that follow and that may or may not indicate cancer. An early visit to the doctor is strongly suggested, since a large percentage of cancer patients can be cured if the disease is discovered at the outset.

- Change in bowel or bladder habits
- A sore that does not heal
- Unusual bleeding or discharge
- Thickening or lump in breast or elsewhere
- Indigestion or difficulty in swallowing

- Obvious change in wart or mole
- Nagging cough or hoarseness

INSPECTING THE THROAT

In infections and communicable diseases, the throat is often one of the first areas to show evidence of illness. Early recognition of a sore throat may help to prevent the spread of disease to other family members. The home nurse should practice throat inspection when family members are well, since each throat appears different. Tonsils vary in size, and the mucous membrane is normally pinkish-red. Thus, changes may be a matter of degree.

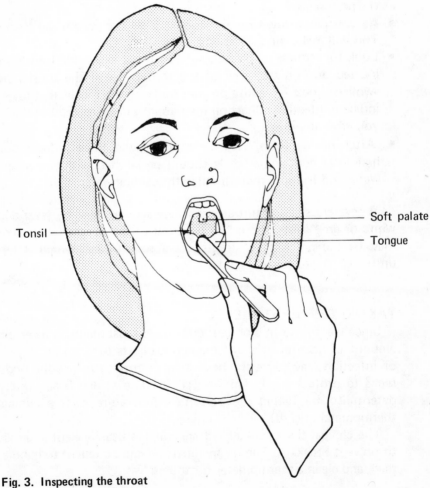

Tonsil —
Soft palate —
Tongue —

Fig. 3. Inspecting the throat

The nurse must be able to see into the back of the patient's throat to examine it properly. Some people are able to lay their tongues flat so that the throat can be easily examined. Others require a tongue depressor or the handle of a spoon (fig. 3). The steps in the procedure are as follows:

- Have the person stand or sit in front of you and tip his head back. You must have sufficient light to see into the back of the throat. A flashlight may be held in one hand and a spoon handle or tongue depressor in the other.
- Place the spoon about two-thirds of the way back on the tongue. Avoid touching the soft palate (uvula), or it will make the person gag.
- As you press down on the spoon, have the person say "Ah." This will make the back cavity wider.
- Look for redness on the sides of the throat where the tonsils are located and on the back of the throat. See if the tonsils are swollen. Look for white or grey spots on the tonsils that might indicate infection. Chart on the patient's daily record the things you have observed.
- After having been used to examine the throat, the spoon handle is contaminated. It should be washed with hot soapy water and friction, then rinsed with scalding water.

A severely swollen throat, especially accompanied by fever and white or grey spots, should be reported to the doctor. Such signs may be indicative of a streptococcal sore throat, which if left untreated, might cause rheumatic fever.

TAKING TEMPERATURE

Since we are warm-blooded, our bodies must maintain a certain amount of heat in order for the various parts to function. Injury or infection may cause the body temperature to rise as the body seeks to protect itself. This rise is called fever and is accurately determined by taking the person's temperature with a clinical thermometer (fig. 4).

The clinical thermometer is fragile and is usually kept in a case to prevent breakage. Family members should be taught to handle, read, and clean a thermometer for themselves.

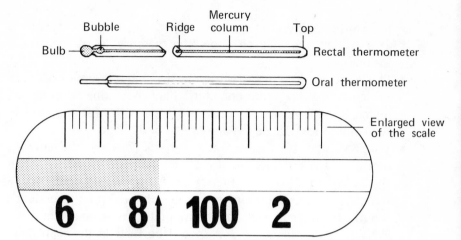

Fig. 4. The clinical thermometer

The parts of the thermometer are as follows:

- The bulb end containing the mercury. A long slender bulb indicates a thermometer that is used for oral (mouth) temperatures. A short stubby bulb, either round or pear-shaped, indicates a thermometer that may be used for taking oral, rectal, or axillary temperatures.

- The bubble near the bulb. It is the constriction that prevents the mercury from going down when it is removed from the person's mouth. It does not prevent the mercury from going up if it is subjected to a higher temperature.

- The scale and ridge against a white background. The scale consists of small lines above the mercury with numbers below. Temperature is read to the nearest two-tenths of a degree.

An arrow indicates the point which is considered an average normal temperature. Clinical thermometers may be marked in either Centigrade or Fahrenheit scale. The Centigrade thermometer goes from 34.5°C to 43.4°C with the arrow at 37°C. The Fahrenheit thermometer scale goes from 94°F to 108°F with the arrow at 98.6°F. With a change to the metric system simply a matter of time, all of us may need at some time to be able to convert one scale to the other. To convert a Centigrade reading to Fahrenheit, multiply the Centigrade reading by 9, divide by 5, and add 32. To convert a Fahrenheit reading to Centigrade, subtract 32 from the Fahrenheit reading, multiply by 5 and divide by 9.

The thermometer is not perfectly round, and the ridge serves as a magnifying area to allow the mercury to be read more easily.

- The mercury column. It is usually silver, but people who have difficulty reading thermometers may buy one with a red mercury column. The mercury expands with heat and rises in the column to indicate the amount of body heat.
- The top end of the thermometer. It never goes into the patient's mouth and is the part handled by the home nurse. Never touch the bulb end with your fingers since that would contaminate the part of the thermometer to be placed into the patient's mouth. In order to read the thermometer, remember that it is a right-handed instrument and should be held in the right hand with the bulb pointing left, the ridge at eye level with the lines above and the numbers below. It may help you to locate the mercury if you look for the bubble and follow the mercury up the column to the point at which it stops.

To use a clinical thermometer observe the following instructions:

- When you are ready to use the thermometer, grasp the top end firmly and remove it from the case.
- Stand away from furniture and shake the thermometer with a loose wrist motion until the mercury is below 96° F.
- Have the patient sit or lie down and ask him to remain there as long as the thermometer is in his mouth.
- Place the thermometer under the patient's tongue and a little to one side and ask him to keep his lips closed around the thermometer. Leave it in position for three minutes.
- Remove the thermometer, wipe it with a tissue, and read it, making sure that you have adequate light to read the mercury accurately.
- Record the reading on the daily record in the appropriate column.
- Clean the thermometer, using the following steps:
  - Hold the thermometer by the top and with a moist, soapy tissue wash the thermometer from top to bottom, using a firm rotating motion. Rinse the thermometer in the sink, using cool, running water, or over a waste container using a dish of cool, clean water.
  - Soap the thermometer a second time in the same way.

- Rinse a second time.
- Dry the thermometer with a dry tissue and replace it in its container, bulb end first. The thermometer should always be cleaned before it is placed in the case.

A rectal temperature is always taken on a small child, on an unconscious or uncooperative patient, or when any condition exists which interferes with breathing. Use a stubby bulb thermometer, lubricate it with vaseline or a water soluble lubricant, and have the patient lie on his side with his knees slightly flexed. Separate the buttocks and insert the thermometer through the rectal sphincter about two inches. The thermometer should be left in place three minutes and should be held by the home nurse so that it will not slip out. Rectal temperatures are very accurate and tend to be about one degree higher than those taken by mouth. Normal average would be about 99.6°F. In recording a rectal temperature, place an R above the number to indicate the method used.　　R

　　99.6°F

A rectal thermometer should be used to take an axillary temperature. The bulb is placed in the armpit (dry the area first if it is moist), and the arm is held snugly against the body for approximately five to ten minutes. Axillary temperature is relatively inaccurate and tends to be about one degree lower with 97.6°F as the average. Axillary temperature is taken when neither oral nor rectal temperature is satisfactory. (Example: a baby with diarrhea.) It is recorded with an A above the number.　　A

　　　　　　　　　　　　　　　　　　　　　　　97.6°F

Special Notes on Taking Temperature

Remember that the normal range of temperature is 97.2°F to 99.4°F and will vary with the time of day and the individual. A cold or other slight infection or dehydration may cause the temperature to rise slightly.

With long-term illnesses, the temperature is usually taken about every four hours during the day, but when a child has a high fever, you may wish to check it more often. When a temperature reaches 104°F or higher, the doctor may instruct you to give the patient a sponge bath or cover him with a towel wrung out of lukewarm water. The evaporation will cool the body, but do not allow the patient to become chilled. Aspirin also helps to reduce fever.

If a patient has had hot or cold liquids in his mouth, wait fifteen to twenty minutes before taking his temperature.

A temperature should be taken whenever a person complains of feeling ill or when there is a sudden change in the patient's condition, such as a chill, restlessness, headache, pain in the chest or the abdomen, sore throat, vomiting, diarrhea, or skin rash. It can be recorded in three ways: 98.6, 98 6/10, or 98^6. Remember to put an R or an A above the number if the temperature was taken by the rectal or axillary method.

If a thermometer should break in a patient's mouth, tell him not to swallow, have him rinse his mouth well, and check his mouth for cuts or glass. If the patient has swallowed glass, notify the doctor and get his advice.

PULSE

Counting the pulse is a method of counting the heartbeat, and there are wide variations in rate even within a single person. The rate may be increased with fever, exercise, fright, or emotional tension. It decreases when a person sleeps. The range is about fifty to ninety beats per minute for a resting heart beat. Usually the person who is in good physical condition has a lower pulse rate. A child's pulse is faster than an adult's, and a woman usually has a faster pulse rate than a man.

The pulse may be taken wherever arteries are near the surface of the skin, such as along the side of the neck or on the thumb side of the wrist. To take the wrist pulse, have the person extend his arm in a relaxed position. Place your three middle fingers along the person's wrist just below his thumb. Press firmly enough to feel the beat. Count the beats for one-half minute and multiply by two to determine the beat for one minute. As you count, be aware of the volume and rhythm. It is not uncommon for a beat to be missed, but a highly irregular pulse should be called to the doctor's attention.

RESPIRATION

Respiration is the process of inhaling and exhaling air. It is the one vital sign over which the patient has some control. It is best to take the respiration while still holding your fingers on the pulse so that the person is not aware that you are counting respirations. Count the pulse during the first half minute, and the respiration during the second half minute. The average respiration rate is sixteen to twenty-four breaths per minute. Notice whether respirations are deep or shallow and whether they are unusually noisy. When fever is present, both pulse and respiration are increased. With a young child, pulse and respiration may be difficult to take, and temperature may be the chief vital sign recorded by the home nurse.

When all three vital signs are taken, they are recorded on the daily record with temperature first, then pulse, then respiration. For example,

T   P   R

102–108–24. Note that if you reversed the temperature and pulse, the doctor would think the patient was in great danger with a temperature of 108; therefore, take care to report accurately.

SUMMARY

The signs and symptoms of illness are the home nurse's guide to further action. The more skilled she is in these areas, the easier it will be for her to make judgments about whether to call the doctor or to wait and see what develops. If possible, the family member should be observed without his knowledge, since he may be tempted to exaggerate his aches and pains in order to receive a little extra attention.

MOVING THE PATIENT

The question of whether to care for a patient at home is a debatable one. What does the patient prefer? Does someone in the family have the time, skill, and emotional stamina to fill the role of home nurse? Does the doctor feel the patient can be cared for at home? Is there an extra room for the patient? How will other family members be affected?

Having weighed the pros and cons, the family must make a decision. Of prime importance once the decision is made is the health of the home nurse. She will need planned relief periodically, supplied by a good-hearted neighbor, another family member, or a hired health professional.

It is well to remember that unless the patient is a child, he will probably be at least as large as the home nurse, and she must be careful not to injure herself in caring for the patient. A knowledge of the principles of good body mechanics can help the home nurse protect herself.

PRINCIPLES OF GOOD BODY MECHANICS FOR THE HOME NURSE

Principles of body mechanics for the home nurse include the following:

- Maintain a broad base of support. Stand with feet slightly apart and one foot ahead of the other. This allows for better balance. Wear comfortable, low-heeled shoes.
- Maintain natural spinal curves. Tighten buttocks and abdominal muscles. This allows for good posture in whatever the home nurse is doing.
- Use certain muscle masses in the body intended for heavy work such as lifting. These muscle masses include the hip and upper leg muscles and the shoulder and upper arm muscles. Yet we often bend our backs to pick up heavy weights. Have you ever noticed that a bushel of peaches or a basket of wet laundry feels very heavy when you start to lift it but seems lighter when you get it up to waist level? The reason is that the small back

muscles are not intended for lifting, and the back protests until the weight is transferred to the leg and shoulder muscles when you stand upright. Even picking up a pencil can cause back injury because you are lifting half your body. Try bending at the knees and hips as you lift a suitcase, a hefty three-year-old, or one edge of the sofa. You will find it is much more comfortable for you.

- Stand near the work area and keep heavy objects as near you as possible. Try holding a basket of wet clothes on your fingertips away from your body. Both your arms and back will complain at the strain. One advantage in having the patient in a single bed is that you are near him regardless of which side of the bed you work from.
- Have the mattress at hip level. This eliminates the need for you, as home nurse, to bend your back excessively in caring for the patient. Perhaps you have attempted to bathe or care for a patient in a bed at the usual height. It is an exceptionally tiring task. Page 147 lists several ways of raising the bed so that the home nurse does not need to bend unnecessarily.
- Roll, slide, turn, or pull the patient. Do not attempt to lift him without adequate help.
- Have the patient help lift himself if he is able, and arrange a signal so that you work together.

BODY MECHANICS FOR THE PATIENT

Body mechanics are just as important for the patient as for the nurse, though the reasons are somewhat different. If you think about it, you will realize that when you don't feel well, you usually curl up in bed. This is not necessarily bad, since you will change your position when your body feels the need. But a person who is too ill to move must be turned by the home nurse every two to four hours. There are several reasons why this is important.

- When the patient remains in one position for long periods of time, contractures form. A contracture is a shortened, deformed muscle, a condition occurring when the muscle is not exercised or moved periodically. It can be prevented by frequent turning and also by exercise. If the patient is unable to move the parts of the body due to paralysis or unconsciousness, the home nurse will probably be instructed by the doctor or physical therapist on how to help him exercise. This is called passive exercise. She will be told how many times a day to perform the exercise and what technique to use.

- Changing positions rests the patient. Those of us who can turn ourselves do this subconsciously. You might think you sleep through the night without moving, but such is not the case. You turn many times during the night. The home nurse must provide this service for the paralyzed, unconscious, or helpless patient.

- Turning helps to prevent bedsores (also called pressure sores or decubitus ulcers). These occur when pressure on a particular area, especially over the bony parts, interferes with the circulation. The base of the spine, the shoulder blades, the heels, and the elbows are commonly involved. First a reddened area occurs. This becomes a greyish-white when pressed and if left uncared for becomes an enlarging, painful sore as the skin breaks away. In addition to turning, other techniques for preventing bed sores include: keeping the bed dry, giving good skin care including adequate back rubs, keeping the bottom sheet tight and smooth, providing adequate nourishment for tissue repair, and using padding of some sort under susceptible areas. A sheepskin under the back and buttocks offers softness, absorbency, natural oil, and air circulation. Although it is difficult to wash, it is an excellent way to help prevent bed sores. A synthetic, furlike material may be used, but it is not absorbent. Foam doughnuts or pads covered with satin may help keep the pressure off heels and elbows. Bed sores are much easier to prevent than to heal.

- Frequent turning helps to keep the body's circulation moving normally. Doctors have learned a great deal about circulation in recent years, and they encourage all types of patients to move about in bed unless instructed otherwise. Frequent movement of the legs is important, since 90 percent of clots form in the legs. Following surgery, patients are asked to cough, deep breathe, and turn as soon as they wake up from the anesthesia. After labor and delivery, women rarely remain in bed more than a few hours. Some people are more prone to circulatory problems than others, and in such people clots occasionally break loose and travel to the lungs or brain, causing further injury or death.

The posture for a patient in bed should include good alignment of body parts and adequate support. Remember to:

- Provide support for the back and joints.
- Watch the extremities to prevent contractures.
- Change the patient's position every two to four hours to increase circulation and prevent pressure sores and contractures.
- Provide passive exercise when necessary to promote good muscle tone.

HELPING THE PATIENT SIT UP

Remember to allow the patient to help himself sit up as much as possible. This provides him with exercise and a feeling of being useful. Be sure you arrange a signal to coordinate his help with yours (fig. 5).

- Have the patient flex his knee.
- Face toward the head of the bed with your outside foot slightly forward.
- Lock near arms with the patient. You grasp his shoulder and he grasps yours.
- Slip your far arm under the patient's neck and shoulders so that his head rests on your forearm.
- On signal, pull back to raise the patient. Steady him until he can sit up without feeling dizzy and until he can brace his hands to support himself.

MOVING A PATIENT TO THE HEAD OF THE BED

Especially in a hospital bed in which the head of the bed can be elevated, a patient tends to slip toward the foot of the bed and must be moved back toward the head of the bed. This may be done in several ways. If the patient can help himself, remove his pillow, flex his knees, have him grasp the head of the bed and pull toward it. You may help by placing your hands under the buttocks to help him slide. You may prefer to help him by using one arm to support his head and shoulders and the other to support his hips. If he is completely helpless and the head board is not too high, you may stand at the head of the bed, reach your hands over the patient's shoulders to grasp his armpits, and pull the patient as you straighten up. This is not a safe procedure, however, for a patient with arthritis or stroke.

MOVING AND TURNING A PATIENT

A single bed is usually too narrow to turn the patient without

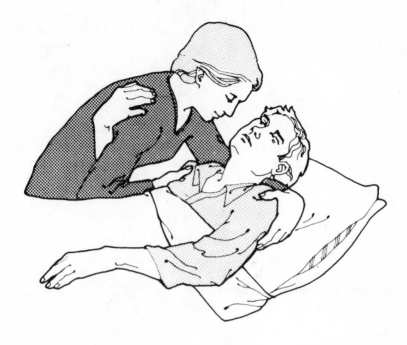

Fig. 5. Helping the patient sit up

pulling him to the edge of the bed first. If he has no severe pain or back involvement, this can be done by moving him in segments. First, place one hand under his head and shoulders and the other hand under his chest. Slide this part of his body toward you. Next, put one hand under his waist and the other under his hips and slide this area. Finally, place one hand under the knees and the other under the ankles and slide his feet and legs. Don't bring the patient too near the edge of the bed.

To turn the patient, cross the ankle near the edge of the bed over his other ankle, then place one of your hands on the patient's hip and one on the patient's shoulder. Roll him onto his side. Flex the patient's upper leg to allow him some support while you position the pillows to brace him (fig. 6).

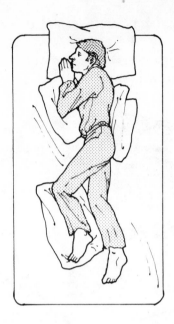

Fig. 6. Bracing a patient with pillows

Sometimes it is impossible to roll a heavy patient unless you go to the other side of the bed and pull him toward you. If you wish to roll the patient over onto his abdomen, be sure his arms are straight at his sides so that no damage will be done to them during the turning process.

USING A DRAWSHEET TO TURN A PATIENT

In the hospital a drawsheet is a long narrow sheet placed across the bed over the bottom sheet. It extends from the patient's shoulders to his knees. It is tucked in along with the bottom sheet. In a home situation a drawsheet can be improvised by folding a regular sheet in half from top to bottom. A drawsheet may be used over a piece of plastic or rubber to protect the bed from any wetness. More often, however, it is used as a turning sheet for a heavy or helpless patient. The one disadvantage is that two or more people are required when a turning sheet is used to move a patient. More instructions for using a turning sheet may be found in the *Red Cross Home Nursing Text.*

PROVIDING COMFORT AND SUPPORT FOR A PATIENT ALLOWED TO SIT UP

As soon as the patient's condition permits, the doctor will allow him to sit up in bed whenever he wishes. This allows the patient more freedom, makes eating easier, facilitates reading and other recreation, and boosts the patient's morale. The first time the patient rises upward, he may become dizzy and weak. The home nurse should supply adequate support. Three pillows positioned to form a pyramid at the head of the bed will offer the most complete support for the patient's back (fig. 7).

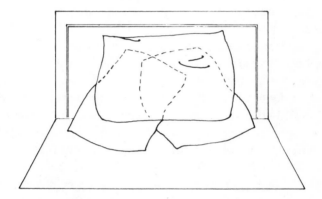

Fig. 7. A pyramid of three pillows as support

If needed, place an extra small support at the patient's lower back and a rolled towel or small blanket under the patient's knees. It is uncomfortable to sit with the legs perfectly straight; however, the knees should not be completely flexed for long periods of time as this may interfere with circulation. A box braced between the foot of the bed and the patient's feet, two inches taller than the patient's toes, will allow his feet to remain in a normal position.

If the patient is allowed to sit up to eat or read, pillows are inadequate and a better back rest will be needed. One can be purchased or improvised by using a card table or board slanted from the headboard. Instructions for the construction of an excellent back rest improvised from a large cardboard box are found on pages 150-51.

A bed table allows the patient to have a solid surface on which to write, play games, or place his meal tray. The bed table is placed on top of the covers, and the home nurse should be sure the bedding is loose enough under the table to allow adequate movement of the patient's legs. A bed table can be made from a cardboard box. (See pages 151-53.)

HELPING THE PATIENT OUT OF BED

Most patients wish to be out of bed as soon as possible since they recognize several advantages:

- They get exercise.
- They feel as if they are getting better.
- They have fewer problems with body elimination.
- They sleep better.
- They feel less of a burden on the home nurse.
- They begin to regain strength.

Usually the doctor allows progressive ambulation, beginning with the patient sitting up in bed. When he tolerates that well, he moves to sitting at the edge of the bed, dangling his legs over the side for short periods of time only. Next, he sits in a chair; and finally he begins to walk about. If the patient has been bedfast for a long period, it may be some time before he has sufficient strength to walk. The home nurse should be on the lookout for dizziness, weakness, and tiredness each time the patient increases his activity.

Before helping the patient out of bed, place a chair parallel to the head or foot of the bed. Help the patient sit up and swing his legs over the edge of the bed. Put on his robe and slippers. If the bed is high, use a footstool. A box or a stack of books or magazines tied together could serve as an improvised footstool. Stand in front of the patient and have him place his hands on your shoulders while you place your hands under his armpits. Support the patient as he steps down. Have him pivot so that he is in front of the chair. If you must support him as you lower him into the chair, step to the side so that you can bend your knees and hips as you lower him into the chair. In helping the patient from the chair to return to bed, use the same technique. This is also a useful technique for helping a weak or arthritic patient in and out of a car. Remember to encourage the patient to help himself whenever possible.

HELPING THE PATIENT TO WALK

When the patient is ready to begin walking, have him wear comfortable, low-heeled shoes. He may be weak and apprehensive, and you should remain close beside him. If he needs support, walk arm-in-arm with him with your hand on top of his (fig. 8). If he becomes weak or faint, you can quickly change hands, your near hand encircling his waist as you broaden your base of support, and lower him to a chair or to the floor if necessary. Don't try to hold him upright if he has fainted since he will regain consciousness only when the blood returns to his brain, and this can occur more quickly if he is lying down.

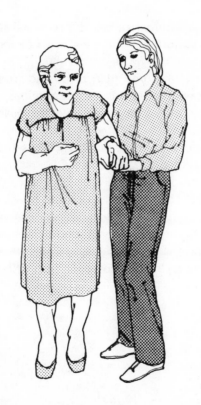

Fig. 8. Helping the patient to walk

In helping a stroke patient (hemiplegic—paralyzed on one side) walk, you should stand on the patient's affected side, with an arm about his waist. This will give him assurance but will not interfere with his balance.

USING A WHEELCHAIR

To prepare a wheelchair for the patient, place it near the foot of the bed. Raise the footrests and set the brakes. Help the patient into the wheelchair as you would into a regular chair. If there is a blanket around him, be sure it will not catch in the wheels. Check to be sure the patient's elbows are inside the arm rests as you go through doors. Pull the chair after you over door sills, into elevators, or off a curb.

SUMMARY

Perhaps we can summarize best by recalling some general principles that are important when we are helping a patient move about:

- Tell the patient what you plan to do and arrange a signal. Even with a patient who appears to be unconscious, it is best to speak to him as you work since he can often hear even though he cannot communicate.
- Allow the patient to do as much for himself as possible unless otherwise instructed by the doctor.
- Change his position frequently, at least every two to four hours.
- Provide support to areas of the body to prevent deformities and discomfort.
- Be aware of the importance of body mechanics for both the home nurse and the patient.
- Never strain yourself. Have someone help when necessary.

THE BEDFAST PATIENT

When a family member is confined to bed twenty-four hours a day, the home nurse must utilize special skills to provide care and comfort. These skills are not difficult and are similar to those used by the professional nurse in the hospital.

ELIMINATION OF WASTES

A bedpan is used by the female for the elimination of body wastes from both the bowel and bladder. The male patient will also need a urinal. Both should be kept covered and preferably out of sight when not in use. The cover should be made of heavy material which has a distinct right and wrong side so that the wrong side of the material is always against the bedpan. A bedpan is a very difficult item to improvise, and one should be borrowed or purchased when the need arises. In handling it, you should avoid touching the open end.

When the patient asks for the bedpan, respond promptly so that he does not have to wait. You may wish to place a pad under the patient to protect the bed. One can be improvised by covering several layers of newspaper with a clean cloth. A metal bedpan is very cold and should be warmed by running warm water into it. Talcum powder sprinkled on the seat of the bedpan will allow it to slide under the patient more easily.

Have the bed flat. Turn back the covers so they neither interfere with nor expose the patient unnecessarily. Have the patient flex her knees so that she can lift her hips when you are ready. A hospital bed equipped with an overhead trapeze bar will make it easier for the patient. Place the pan cover nearby. Slide one hand under the patient's back while holding the pan with your other hand. On signal use your hand as a lever to help her lift her hips as you slide the pan under her. The open end should point between the patient's legs and the rounded part should fit snugly under the buttocks. The patient will probably be more comfortable if she can have her head raised at least slightly. This position also allows the patient's bowel and bladder to empty more easily with the aid of gravity. Three pillows or a backrest may be positioned for her to use. Before leaving the room, adjust the bed covers and be sure the patient is comfortable and has access to a roll of toilet paper and some means of calling you when she is through. Do not be gone long. When you are ready to remove the pan, reposition the patient flat on her back with her knees flexed. Help the patient clean herself if necessary. Be sure her hips are raised high enough so that the skin does not adhere to the pan as it is removed. Cover the pan. Adjust the patient's position and offer her soap and water so that she may wash her hands. Observe the contents of the bed pan for any abnormalities before emptying it into the toilet. Rinse the pan with cold water to prevent fecal material from sticking; then wash the inside thoroughly with warm, soapy water and a toilet brush. Cover the pan and return it to the bedside. When the procedure is completed, be sure you wash your hands, then record the appropriate information on the patient's daily record.

To give a bedpan to a very helpless or heavy patient, roll her on her side, place the pan against the buttocks, and hold it snugly while the patient rolls back onto the bedpan. When the patient is ready to roll off the bedpan, be very careful that the pan does not tip. If the patient needs help in rolling, one person should roll her while another holds the bedpan steady.

If a patient has difficulty starting to urinate, the sound of running water or warm water poured over the genitals may help. Sometimes the home nurse is instructed to measure the urinary output and record it on the daily record. She would also need to measure and record the patient's liquid intake.

Doctors realize that very few patients enjoy using a bedpan, and whenever possible they allow bathroom privileges. If the patient is very weak, a commode chair may be used at the bedside, thus eliminating the trip to the bathroom. The commode may be made from an old wooden chair with a hole cut in the center of the seat. It allows the patient to sit in a normal position for body elimination and therefore requires much less effort on her part.

Because of inactivity, more bland diet, and a prone or supine position, it is not unusual for the bedfast patient to be plagued by constipation. If he dislikes using the bedpan, he may put off having to use it, thus encouraging further constipation. Under normal conditions food is carried through the digestive tract by wave-like movements called peristalsis. The food nutrients are extracted in the small bowel, and excess water is absorbed in the large bowel. The longer the waste material remains in the large bowel, the more water is extracted. After several days the fecal material may become hard and compact and difficult to expel from the body. The home nurse can help by encouraging the patient to consume adequate fluid to have regular bowel habits, and to eat plenty of fruits and vegetables. If constipation continues, the doctor may recommend an enema, a laxative, or a suppository to relieve the problem. Disposable enema units which are quick and easy to use can be purchased at the drugstore. Simply follow the instructions given. This is the easiest way to give an enema to a young child or an older adult who may have difficulty retaining large amounts of fluid.

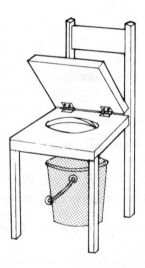

Fig. 9. Bedside commode chair

MOUTH CARE

We discussed on page 3 the necessity of good dental hygiene in preventing dental decay. The bedfast patient must have an opportunity to clean and refresh his mouth. If he is able to sit up in bed, it is simply a matter of placing his equipment, a glass of water, and a small basin on the overbed table so that he can carry out the procedure.

For the helpless patient who must remain lying down, use the following steps:

- Place a towel under the patient's head and one under his chin.
- Turn his head to the side and place a small basin (called an emesis basin in the hospital. A sardine can or other fairly flat receptable will work well) near his chin.
- Brush the patient's teeth for him and allow him to suck water through a straw to rinse his mouth. He can spit the water into the basin.

An unconscious patient also needs frequent mouth care because his mouth tends to remain open while he breathes and the air going in and out creates smelly crusts called sordes on the mucous membranes. About every two hours, perhaps each time you turn the patient, use the following procedure:

- Place a towel over the pillow.
- Moisten a large applicator with a salt and soda solution (½ tsp. of each in a glass of water). Press the applicator on the side of the glass to get rid of excess solution. No moisture should be allowed to drip into the unconscious patient's throat.
- Steady the patient's chin and swab all areas of the mouth including the tongue and teeth. Change applicators when necessary.
- Apply lubricant to the patient's lips to prevent cracking.

If the patient has dentures and is conscious, give him a tissue to remove them and hand them to you. Dentures are most easily cleaned under running water. If your experience with dentures is limited, be careful; they are slippery and may chip if dropped. Place a washcloth in the bottom of the wash basin so that if they slip from your hand as you clean them, they will not be damaged. When they are clean, return them to the patient in a cup of water. It is easier for the patient to insert them into his mouth if they are moist. If the patient does not wish to wear his dentures, check with the dentist for appropriate instructions as to their care when stored.

THE BATH

Although many people consider a daily bath a necessity, the home nurse should remember that a partial bath may sometimes suffice for the patient. A complete bath is very tiring and may cause excessive dryness, especially with an elderly person. On the other hand, a bath cleans, refreshes, helps get rid of waste products from the skin, aids circulation, and provides both passive and active exercise. Only those patients who are acutely ill, helpless, or confined to bed should have a bed bath; and even then, the patient should be encouraged to do as much for himself as possible.

Any time of day is acceptable as bath time. It depends on the patient's desires and the nurse's time schedule. You will need about 45 minutes to an hour to do the bath, the back rub, the bed change, and straighten the room. Before beginning the procedure, make sure the room is warm, that all equipment is available, and that you will not be unnecessarily interrupted. Equipment includes a basin of warm water (to be changed when it gets cool, soapy, or dirty), a washcloth, two bath towels, and soap in a soap dish (never allow soap to remain in the wash basin). The steps of the procedure are these:

- Remove the top covers and cover the patient with a sheet blanket (called a bath blanket). A sheet blanket is warmer and more absorbent and will allow you to reuse the top sheet. If the patient is chilly, place a hot water bottle at his feet.
- Remove the patient's gown or pajamas and place a dry towel over the pillow under his head.
- Make a bath mitt (fig. 10) to prevent dripping water on the patient.

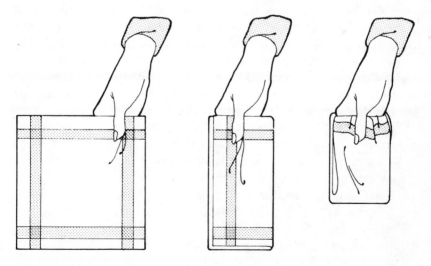

Fig. 10. Bath mitt

- Wash the eyes gently from the nose outward, using a separate corner of the washcloth for each eye (fig. 11).

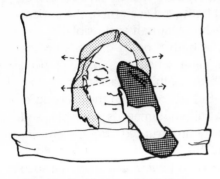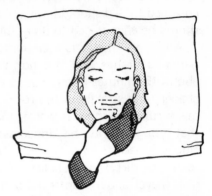

Fig. 11. Bathing a patient's face

- Wash the entire face: forehead, nose, cheeks, and under chin. Use soap only if the patient desires it. Wrap a corner of the towel around your hand and dry the face. Never cover the patient's face with the towel as most people feel smothered when their faces are covered.
- Wash the neck and ears; rinse and dry.
- Remove the towel from under the patient's head and place it over the patient's chest. Pull the bath blanket down to the abdomen. Soap, rinse and dry the chest, working under the towel. Pay special attention to the areas under the breasts where irritation may occur. Wash, rinse, and dry the abdomen, working under the bath blanket. Remember that many people are ticklish in this area. Use long smooth strokes to prevent a tickling sensation. Replace the bath blanket and remove the towel.
- Place one towel under the patient's near arm and the second towel over the arm. Soap, rinse, and dry, and remember to do the armpit (axilla). Place the basin on the bed and allow the patient to place her hand in the water while you wash it.
- Follow the same procedure for the far arm. Hopefully, this can be done without having to move all the equipment to the other side of the bed. Be sure to replace the bath blanket over each area after it is dried.
- Expose the near leg and place the towel under it. Be careful not to expose the genital area. Wash, rinse, and dry the leg. Place the basin on the bed, have the patient flex her knee and place

her foot in the basin. This is an excellent way to soak the toenails to facilitate cutting them. In elderly people the toenails become very thick and brittle, difficult to cut unless they have been soaked.

- Follow the same procedure for the far leg. Change the water before proceeding.
- Turn the patient on her side and placing the towel parallel to her back, soap, rinse, and dry. Use alcohol or lotion to give a back rub. (See next section.) Turn patient onto her back.
- Put a towel under the patient's buttocks. If she is able, place all equipment within her reach and allow her to wash the genital area. If she cannot do it, you must do it for her. This area becomes very sore and irritated if left unwashed.
- Remove the bath equipment and help the patient put on her pajamas.
- If the patient is difficult to turn, wash the genital area (step 13), then turn the patient on her side to wash her back and do a back rub. Proceed with the bed making. One extra turn is eliminated.

BACK RUB

A back rub stimulates circulation, refreshes and relaxes the patient, and helps to prevent bedsores from developing. The home nurse should inspect the skin surfaces of the back carefully and give special attention to any reddened areas.

The equipment needed includes lotion or alcohol. To take the chill off the liquid, place the bottle in a pan of warm water for a few minutes. Alcohol is drying, but will cool the skin effectively. The home nurse should consider whether alcohol or lotion meets her patient's needs better.

The steps in the procedure fit into the bath routine after the back is washed. A back rub in the evening is usually part of preparing the patient for sleep. Two back rubs a day are a minimum for a bedfast patient.

- Position the patient on his side or abdomen near the edge of the bed where you are standing.
- Be sure a towel is under the patient's back and buttocks to protect the bed.
- Face the head of the bed with your outer foot slightly forward. This allows you to rock back and forth as you rub the back.

- Pour lotion or alcohol into your hands. Be sure your hands are warm before you begin. Your nails should be short, and you should avoid rings with large settings.
- Place your hands at the base of the spine with your fingers pointing in the direction of the neck. Use heavy pressure as you move up the spine to the neck and lighter pressure as you move outward over the shoulders and downward toward the buttocks. Keep your hands lubricated and use a swinging rhythmic motion to help relax the patient. Continue the back rub for three to five minutes. Kneading the area near the neck and shoulders may reduce tiredness and tension in that area. Where reddened areas are noticed, do additional circular massage. Reddened areas are particularly apt to occur at the base of the spine and on the shoulder blades.

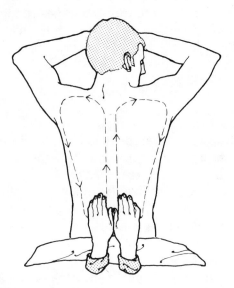

Fig. 12. The back rub

BED MAKING

It is always easier to make the bed when the patient is sitting in a chair or while he is taking a tub bath. Sometimes, however, the patient is bedfast, and changing the bed linen is a bit tricky for the novice. Let us consider the best method to be used. Bed making usually follows the completion of the bath, and the home nurse should have clean linens ready before she begins. Bedding should be changed as necessary and does not need to be changed every day as long as it remains dry, clean, tight, and smooth. A clean, tight bed not only provides comfort for the patient, but helps to prevent bedsores.

The procedure is as follows:

- Have the patient roll to the far side of the bed. He does not need to be teetering on the edge, however, since you really need only a small space for spreading out the bottom sheet.
- Loosen the bedding along the side. Remember that the top bedding was removed before you began the bath, and the patient has a bath blanket over him for warmth.
- Gather the edge of the sheet and push it toward the patient's back, bunching it closely against him under the bath blanket (fig. 13).

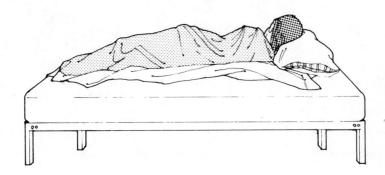

Fig. 13. Making the bed around the patient

- Place a clean sheet, lengthwise and right side up, on the bed, allowing eighteen inches at the top of the mattress. The bottom edge of the sheet will come just to the bottom edge of the mattress. Center the sheet next to the patient and allow the side of the sheet to hang over the edge of the bed.
- Look at figure 14 and follow it to learn how to make a square corner at the head of the bed. First, tuck the top width of the sheet under the head of the mattress. Then grasp the sheet at point A and raise it up to form a triangle. Lay this triangle back

on the bed while you tuck in the hanging portion of the sheet. Using the palm of your hand to hold the sheet in place, drop point A. Remove your hand and tuck the sheet in all along the side to the foot of the bed.

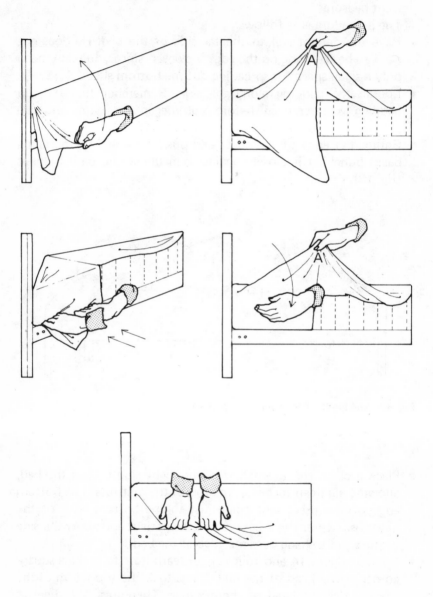

Fig. 14. Squaring the corner of the sheet

- Have the patient roll toward you. Reach behind him and push the bunched sheets toward the far side of the bed. The patient may remain on his side or may lie on his back while you go to the other side of the bed to complete the placement of the bottom sheet.
- Remove the soiled sheet and place with other soiled linens. Smooth out the clean sheet. Proceed as before to tuck the top of the sheet in and make a square corner.
- Beginning near the square corner, gather the sheet in your hands and pull, bracing your knee against the bed. As you pull each area, tuck it under the mattress while you continue to maintain tension on it. This will make the sheet tight and smooth (fig. 15).

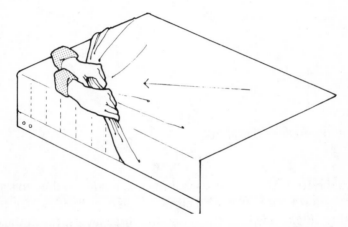

Fig. 15. Pulling the sheet tight

A contour sheet may be used and will eliminate the need for making square corners and tightening the bottom sheet. It will remain smooth longer but will wear out faster because of the added tension caused by the contouring. A contour sheet is placed on the bed in the same way as a regular sheet when the patient is in the bed.

- Next, replace the top sheet wrong side up over the bath blanket. Ask the patient to grasp the top of the sheet while you pull the bath blanket out toward the foot of the bed. Center and position the sheet and make a four-inch cuff under the patient's chin.

- Place the blanket over the sheet with the top edge under the cuff of the sheet.
- Add a bedspread if desired. Bring the top of the spread up over the top of the blanket to protect the blanket. This allows the blanket to be covered by both the spread and the cuff of the sheet (fig. 16).

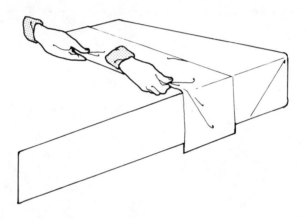

Fig. 16. Protecting the blanket

- At the foot of the bed a pleat may be made to allow toe space. Make a square corner with all three layers of bedding. Go to the other side of the bed, straighten the three layers, finish the cuff, and make a square corner (fig. 17).

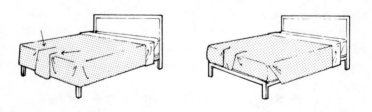

Fig. 17. Making a pleat for toe space

- If the patient cannot stand the weight of the covers on his feet, make a cradle out of a cardboard box (see instructions in chapter twelve for an overbed table) and place it over his feet. Bring the covers over the box and tuck them in or pin them neatly to hold them in place.
- The pillowcase may be the most contaminated part of the bedding, since it contains discharges from the nose and throat. Never place the pillow between your teeth or under your chin when working with it. The pillowcase can be removed by pushing the case off with your wrists as you work your hands up the pillow. To put on the clean pillowcase, turn it inside out and place one hand in each corner of the case, grasp the pillow and flip the case off your hands onto the pillow. Pull the pillowcase down over the pillow (fig. 18). Position the pillow under the patient's head and neck.

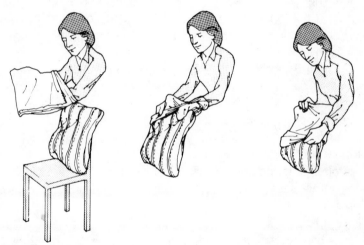

Fig. 18. Putting a clean pillowcase on a pillow

- Remove the soiled linen.

HAIR AND SKIN CARE
Points to remember:
- Fingernails and toenails should be kept trimmed and short.
- Corns and calluses should not be trimmed with a razor blade or a knife. A cut on the feet or legs is often slow to heal, particularly in patients with circulatory problems or diabetes.
- Male patients should be shaved when necessary. It is easier for

the home nurse if she uses an electric razor, since she is not so apt to nick the patient.

- The hair should be arranged simply and should be brushed often enough to prevent snarling. Braids or pony tails will help to keep long hair away from the back of the head.
- If the patient cannot have his hair washed, use dry shampoo to help remove oil. Cotton balls moistened with alcohol or corn meal rubbed lightly into the scalp will also help remove excess oil. Help the patient to understand that his hair is not damaged if he cannot wash it as often as he is used to.
- Instructions for giving a bed patient a shampoo can be found in the *Red Cross Home Nursing* textbook. A bed shampoo should not be given without a doctor's permission.

EQUIPMENT LEFT AT THE BEDSIDE

When the bath procedure is finished, the home nurse should straighten up the room and make the patient comfortable. When the home nurse leaves the room, she should be sure the patient has access to the following items:

- A call bell of some kind. Two lids, a spoon and glass of water, a whistle, or a New Year's Eve noisemaker may be used if you have no bell available.
- Tissue wipes or handkerchiefs.
- A waste container such as a newspaper sack or grocery bag pinned to the bed.
- A pitcher of liquid and a glass. Having extra liquid in the pitcher allows the patient to help himself without calling the nurse. Remember that we should encourage the patient to drink plenty of liquid.
- A bed bag for small articles. This should be about 12 by 20 inches. The piece that goes under the mattress should form a pocket into which a piece of cardboard can be inserted to provide stability for the bed bag (fig. 19; see chapter eleven for further instructions).
- Recreation materials according to the age and interest of the patient.

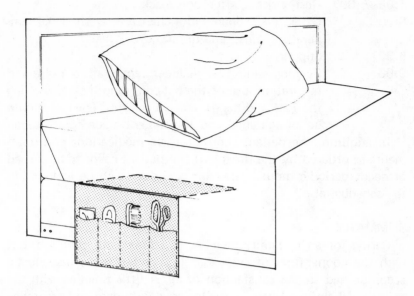

Fig. 19. Providing stability for the bed bag

TYPICAL DAILY SCHEDULE OF ACTIVITIES IN THE SICK ROOM

7:00–8:00   Morning care.—This includes taking the temperature, pulse, and respiration, offering the patient the bedpan, washing his face and hands, doing mouth care, and smoothing the bed. It may also include shaving the patient and combing his hair. Remember that unless ordered otherwise by the doctor, the patient should be allowed to do as many of these things for himself as he can.

8:00–9:00   Breakfast and rest.

9:00–10:00   Offer the bedpan, complete the bath and the back rub, change the bed, and position the patient comfortably. Allow a mid-morning snack if desired.

11:30   Offer the bedpan and give the patient a chance to wash his face and hands. Take temperature, pulse, and respiration.

12:00   Lunch.

1:00—5:00	Rest, visitors, afternoon snack.
5:00	Offer the bedpan and a chance to wash. Take temperature, pulse, and respiration.
5:30	Supper.
9:00	Evening care. This includes temperature, pulse and respiration, use of the bedpan, mouth care, washing the face and hands, and a back rub. The bed should be straightened and the patient made comfortable.

In addition, the patient should receive medications and treatments as ordered by the doctor. If the patient needs to be turned or needs periodic mouth care, this would need to be included in the schedule also.

SUMMARY

Caring for an ill family member is a time-consuming job, but with the cooperation of every family member it can usually be accomplished to the satisfaction of all. A little practice with the skills will help the home nurse to move with ease and assurance and will help the patient to relax and concentrate on getting better. If the home nurse needs help with special procedures, she should contact the local public health office and arrange for a nurse to come to the home and teach her the necessary skills.

DIET DURING ILLNESS

Earlier we included good nutrition as one of the ways we can help to prevent illness among family members. We talked about the basic four food groups and the need to plan menus around these foods. When illness occurs, food still remains an important consideration because it provides the essential nutrients for body repair. Sometimes the doctor expects the home nurse to know how to modify the diet to suit the needs of the patient. At other times he may give her specific instructions and printed materials to help her plan special diets.

Let us consider in this chapter the liquid and soft diets often used during minor illnesses even when the home nurse does not consult the doctor.

A CLEAR LIQUID DIET

Usually foods and liquids are withheld for a few hours during an acute attack of vomiting or diarrhea. However, the home nurse should remember that small children dehydrate quickly when there is excessive loss of body fluids. Severe dehydration can cause death and is evidenced by lack of urine production and lack of saliva in the mouth. Vomiting is usually limited to a few hours after which the discomfort moves lower in the digestive tract, creating cramps and diarrhea. Regardless of whether the problem is due to food poisoning, flu, colds or throat infections, the treatment is to put the digestive tract at rest while preventing dehydration. This can best be done by using a clear liquid diet. A clear liquid diet is one that is transparent and contains no residue. Fruit and vegetable juices would need to be strained to fit in this category. Clear broth, bouillon, and consommé are all clear liquids as are carbonated beverages, Tang, Kool-Aid, and other forms of soft drinks. Tea may be used. One problem with a clear liquid diet is the sameness—all liquids. Substances which are in solid form when eaten but become clear liquids at body temperature allow some variety for the patient. These would include jello, honey, hard candies, all-day suckers, and popsicles (or other ices). Popsicles are of particular value in getting a child with a sore throat to take fluids. No milk products may be used on a clear liquid diet.

A clear liquid diet is impossible to balance nutritionally since it lacks proteins, roughage, and perhaps some vitamins and minerals. Fortunately, it is normally used for only a few days while the digestive tract is recovering; so good nutrition is not its main objective. It is often used in the hospital following abdominal surgery.

The home nurse may wish to make the quantity of liquid more acceptable to the patient by serving six meals a day instead of three.

A FULL LIQUID DIET

While a clear liquid diet is usually a temporary measure, a full liquid diet may be necessary for a prolonged period of time, as in the case of a broken jaw which has been wired shut, or an unconscious patient, fed through a tube. Babies, of course, begin life on a full liquid diet, and some doctors use it during acute ulcer attacks. Fortunately, with a little planning, this diet can provide all the necessary nutrients. Most foods can be liquified by using a blender or a strainer and adding additional liquid. Let's see how we can use foods from each of the four food groups to make a full liquid diet.

- *Milk group:* Much of the protein in a full liquid diet comes from milk products. Ice cream, malts, sodas, and eggnogs are well tolerated by most patients. Extra protein can be furnished by adding additional powdered milk to milk dishes. Cream soups, sherbets, and junket can be used.
- *Meat group—including meat and eggs:* Eggs can be used in thin custards and eggnogs. Meat dishes such as spaghetti and meatballs can be put in the blender with additional broth, bouillon, or tomato juice. Baby meat can also be used by adding broth. Soups can be run through the blender to break up the larger particles.
- *Bread-cereal group:* Gruel can be made with cereal and increased milk or water. Noodles or crackers in soup will break up in the blending process.
- *Vegetables and fruit group:* Juices of both fruits and vegetables may be used. Cream soups run through the blender will help add adequate vegetables to the diet.

All substances used in the clear liquid diet can also be used in the full liquid diet, but remember that such things as carbonated beverages and popsicles add little in food value. Once again the patient will probably prefer six meals a day rather than four or five glasses of different liquids for each meal as would be necessary on a three-meal-a-day plan.

A SOFT DIET

A soft diet is modified so that it is easy to digest and leaves little residue in the digestive tract. This means that seeds, skins, fibers, raw foods, fried foods, and spicy foods are eliminated. Sometimes a soft diet means literally "soft" as for a patient who has had teeth removed and cannot chew satisfactorily. Normally, a soft diet may include such hard substances as toast, crackers, crisp bacon, or tender steak since these are all easy to digest.

SPECIAL DIETS

For a special diet the home nurse usually receives material telling her which foods to include and which to exclude. With diseases such as diabetes, ulcers, colitis, and many others, diet is a vitally important part of the long-term treatment, and the home nurse should learn all she can about how to implement the special diet. Sometimes a patient needs a great deal of support in making drastic changes in eating habits. When cardiac patients first try low-salt foods or foods in which salt substitutes are used, they are sure that they will never be able to make the adjustment.

RULES FOR PREPARING MEALS FOR PATIENTS

- Allow the patient to use the bedpan and to wash before the meal is served. Then be sure he is positioned comfortably to eat.
- Remember that the patient is not exercising and may not need as much food as when he is up and about. See that what he eats (without force) includes the basic nutrients.
- Food plays an important part in all our lives, and patients usually look forward to meals. Have a schedule and adhere to it so that he does not have to wait.
- Appearance is important. Make the tray attractive and include a card or favor or a joke cut from a magazine.
- Make the servings small unless the patient has an increased appetite. Include plenty of liquids.

- Season food to the patient's taste unless diet restrictions preclude this. Use foods the patient likes when possible.
- Be sure that hot foods are hot and cold foods are cold.
- Have another family member eat in the same room with the patient if possible.
- Remove the tray promptly when the patient is through.
- Chart on the daily record the type of diet and the amounts eaten if out of the ordinary.

PLANNING MENUS

Obviously the home nurse will save time if she does not have to fix separate meals for the ill family member. To prevent this she must use care in planning her menus. The clear liquid diet is difficult to adapt from regular menus but does not involve much preparation. Let's look at a sample menu which would be well balanced and could be modified for a soft or full liquid diet.

	Regular Diet	Soft Diet	Full Liquid Diet
BKFST 8:00 a.m.	Oatmeal Orange Toast & Jam Milk	Oatmeal Orange juice Toast & butter Milk	Oatmeal gruel Orange juice Milk
10:00 a.m.			Eggnog

LUNCH	Toasted cheese
	  sandwich
	Cream of asparagus
	  soup
	
	Tomatoes
	Stirred custard
		Toasted cheese
		  sandwich
		Cream of asparagus
		  soup
		
		Tomato juice
		Stirred custard
			
			Cream of asparagus
			  soup (run through
			  the blender)
			Tomato juice
			Stirred custard

3:00 p.m.			Fruit juice

DINNER	Swiss steak
	
	Mashed potatoes
	  & gravy
	Green beans
	Fruit pie a la mode
		Swiss steak
		
		Mashed potatoes
		  & butter
		Green beans
		Ice cream
			Baby meat with added
			  broth
			Liquified potatoes
			  & hot milk
			Liquified green beans
			Ice cream

8:00 p.m.			Milk shake

FEEDING THE ONE WHO IS ILL

A sick child is apt to be fussy about his food. Encourage him to take adequate liquids, but don't worry too much about solid foods. If his appetite is slow to return, utilize his favorite foods, use small portions, and have a little surprise with each meal. Also be creative in the way foods are offered. A small baked potato on toothpick legs with a marshmallow head makes a delectable animal.

For an elderly family member who is ill, meals must continue to meet nutritional needs. Remember that food likes and dislikes are established when one is quite young, and an older person may not care for newer types of food. Many older people have never developed a taste for frozen orange juice, T.V. dinners, and lasagna, though they may relish an orange, meat and potatoes, or spaghetti and meatballs. Some older people have problems with their teeth or dentures, and foods may need to be modified or dental work may need to be done. A loss in the sense of smell in older people may also diminish their enjoyment of food.

During all of our adult life nutritional needs remain fairly constant, though the need for calories may diminish somewhat during latter years. Adequate protein for repair of tissues, necessary vitamins and adequate minerals, especially iron and calcium, are very important in the diet of older people. Sometimes fats are cut down or changed in type due to problems with cholesterol. We have already mentioned that the bedfast patient requires less energy and so should have fewer calories.

When the patient is too weak to feed himself, this task falls to the home nurse or some other family member. It is not an easy job because the patient feels embarrassed by his lack of independence. It is often hard to know how fast to feed him or in what sequence. You might wish to experiment with family members who are well, allowing them to feed each other at the supper table. They will gain empathy very quickly for both the patient and the home nurse. Keep in mind the following rules:

- Make sure the patient is comfortable. Have his head elevated unless it is against the doctor's orders.
- Protect the bedding, and allow him to hold a napkin if he has the use of one of his hands. Place a towel under his chin.
- Sit down by the patient, be unhurried, talk to him, and allow him to do as much as he can for himself.

- Be sure hot foods will not burn him. They can be tested by dropping a little on your wrist. It should sting but not redden the skin.

If the patient is on a liquid diet and especially if he must remain flat, the home nurse will find that using a straw is most acceptable to the patient because it allows him to control the flow of the liquids. The technique is as follows:

- Stir the liquid to distribute the heat evenly.
- Place the glass at the side of the patient's head and have him turn toward it.
- Hold the straw steady as he sucks from it. He may be able to hold it for himself.
- Be sure the straw is below the level of the liquid so that he does not swallow air.
- When the patient has finished, rinse the straw with water if it is to be reused.

Sometimes a patient is too weak to suck through a straw and needs to be fed liquids from a spoon. The procedure is as follows:

- Position the patient comfortably and protect the bedding.
- Hold the cup or bowl near him as you feed him.
- Test the temperature of hot liquids on your wrist.
- Fill the spoon 2/3 full and remove any drips from the bottom of the spoon. Point the bowl of the spoon toward you as you move the spoon toward the patient.
- Touch the patient's lower lip as a signal for him to open his mouth before you tip the spoon. This is particularly useful in feeding a blind patient since it prevents his feeling like a baby bird who must hold his mouth open all the time in order not to miss a spoonful.

Sometimes a patient may have his head lifted up only briefly to swallow something such as medicine. Many people cannot swallow pills while they are lying down. The home nurse should put the pill in the patient's mouth, reach under his head and shoulders, and raise him up with one hand while holding the cup to his lips. If he can help, allow him to control the flow of liquid by tipping the cup.

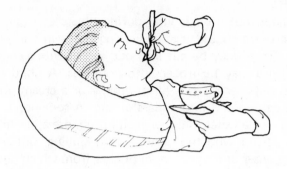

Fig. 20. Touching the patient's lower lip

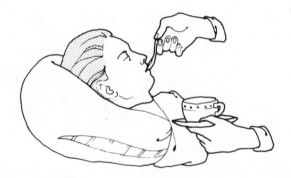

Fig. 21. Tipping the spoon

CARE OF DISHES

Remember that food which has been in the patient's room is contaminated and should not be used by other family members. The dishes from the sick room should be washed with hot, soapy water and plenty of friction and should be rinsed with scalding water. Allow them to air dry before reusing. Where isolation technique is necessary, disposable paper plates, cups, napkins, and plastic utensils are helpful.

SUMMARY

Since good nutrition is vital during illness and convalescence, the home nurse should use all her ingenuity in perking up poor appetites. Bread may be cut into odd shapes with a cookie cutter, or fruit juice may be frozen into popsicles. A child may enjoy having his milk served in a syrup pitcher or a cream pitcher from which he can pour it into a glass or cup. A soda-pop bottle and a straw may make water, milk, or fruit juice more appealing.

For a person who has trouble with spilling, put liquids in a catsup dispenser or a small cream pitcher from which he can drink.

Don't make the tray too crowded. Serve the dessert separately if necessary, and remove the tray promptly when the patient has finished. Soft music may add to the atmosphere if a patient must remain in bed to eat.

MEDICATIONS AND TREATMENTS

In recent years doctors and other scientists have discovered many wonderful and valuable medicines that can help to relieve suffering and cure illness. All of us at one time or another have benefited from these discoveries, but we need to be aware that while medicines may be life-saving, they may also be dangerous when taken unwisely. We should make it a rule to use medications only under the guidance of a doctor or other health personnel and then only when necessary and in the prescribed amounts. It is true that some illnesses such as diabetes, heart disease, high blood pressure, and others may require regular daily medication for many years. On the other hand, many people have become overly dependent on nonprescription drugs to put them to sleep, wake them up, remove minor aches and pains, ease tension, provide elimination, and get them through the day. Sociologists tell us that one of the reasons for the drug culture among young people is their awareness of adult dependence on drugs.

COMMON TYPES OF MEDICINES USED IN THE HOME

- Pain relievers of various kinds are found in almost every home. Aspirin is the least expensive, and if family members find it effective, you may wish to keep a supply on hand. All aspirin contains the same amount of pain reliever whether it is a name brand or not. The more expensive brands have better inert ingredients holding the tablet together, and if you are storing the medicine for a period of time, these tablets would be less apt to break up.

Aspirin comes in five-grain tablets, and two tablets is considered an average adult dose. Below is a table for children. Most children's medicines are based on the weight of the child. A child who is small for his age may need slightly less aspirin than listed.

Give Every Four Hours

Age of child	Tempra Syrup	Baby Aspirin (1¼-grain tablets)
Birth to 6 months	¼ teaspoon	¼ - ½ tablet
6 months to 1 year	½ teaspoon	½ tablet
1 to 2 years	1 teaspoon	1 tablet
2 to 3 years	1 teaspoon	2 tablets
3 to 4 years	2 teaspoons	3 tablets
4 to 5 years	2 teaspoons	4 tablets
Over 5 years	2 teaspoons	1 adult tablet (5 grains)
10 years		2 adult tablets (10 grains)

Ringing in the ears usually indicates that the patient is taking too much aspirin.

Some aspirin compounds have added ingredients such as caffeine to make the aspirin more effective. They are much more expensive than aspirin, but some family members may find that they work better. Buffered aspirin has a substance to counteract stomach acidity caused by aspirin. Family members who have an upset stomach after taking aspirin may wish to take the aspirin with milk or a cracker.

- Laxatives are used by many people—often needlessly. Adequate exercise, plenty of roughage, and a good supply of liquids will usually solve the problem. Health professionals assure us that a daily bowel movement is not necessary, yet we are besieged with TV commercials of weary, headachy people whose only problem is "irregularity." Doctors rarely prescribe laxatives and usually seek to find the source of the constipation instead. It is true, however, that certain conditions tend to induce constipation. Bedfast patients may have problems in this area. Children may become constipated when traveling long distances by car. They lack exercise and adequate fluids and often eat hamburgers and french fries as their main menu day after day.

  The home nurse does not need to contact the doctor to administer a laxative occasionally, but she should check with him before allowing a family member to take laxatives regularly. There are four main types of laxatives, all of which are available without a prescription:

  - Lubricant laxatives, such as mineral oil, simply lubricate the digestive tract. Mineral oil, however, absorbs fat-soluble vitamins as it moves through the digestive tract and so should be used only rarely.

- Bulk-forming cathartics (another term for laxative) are made of cellulose, which swells and adds bulk to the stool. Metamucil is an example of this type. The effect is slow and may not be noticed for twelve to seventy-two hours.

- Chemical cathartics actually stimulate peristalsis and can cause cramping, discomfort, and diarrhea if taken in large quantities. Castor oil and most over-the-counter laxatives fit into this category.

- Saline cathartics work by retaining extra water in the lower bowel, causing the expulsion of fecal material. The most well known of these is Milk of Magnesia.

- Antibiotics are usually obtained by prescripton, but the home nurse should understand certain principles when she gives them to a family member.

  - Antibiotics are truly miracle drugs and have saved millions of lives around the world, especially among children, but they do sometimes have severe side effects and should not be used except under the direction of health personnel.

  - Indiscriminate taking of antibiotics tends to develop drug-resistant strains of bacteria, and scientists have had to seek new types of antibiotics as new forms of bacteria develop. Sometimes people do not take antibiotics for fear they will develop a resistance to them. It is the bacteria that becomes resistant, not the people.

  - Remember that most antibiotics are effective only against bacteria, not viruses, so asking the doctor for a shot of penicillin every time you have a cold or flu is useless, since both of these illnesses are caused by viruses.

  - Antibiotics work by inhibiting the bacteria, and this takes time. The symptoms may disappear in twenty-four to forty-eight hours, but many bacteria continue to linger in the system. The patient should continue to take the medicine as long as directed, usually ten to fourteen days in the case of upper respiratory infections.

- Cold remedies. Since colds are caused by viruses, there is no known cure. There is an old saying, "A cold lasts seven days if you treat it and a week if you don't." Hence, cold remedies can do nothing more than provide temporary relief from certain cold symptoms. If you find one that helps you in this respect, use it, but remember that some cold remedies, especially those with antihistamines, may cause sleepiness or other side effects.

- Vitamin and mineral supplements. This is another highly advertised form of medication, and many homemakers administer supplements to family members "just to be on the safe side." We know that certain vitamins and minerals are stored in the body, and excesses could be dangerous. Other vitamins are simply excreted when taken in excess so that we are wasting our money by taking extra amounts. With a little knowledge of nutrition and food preparation, every homemaker can guarantee adequate vitamin and mineral intake in the meals she serves. For special conditions the doctor may prescribe vitamin and mineral supplements, and the home nurse should encourage the patient to follow the doctor's instructions.
- Assorted over-the-counter drugs, including diet pills, pep pills, and sleeping pills. Most of these medications contain smaller amounts of medicine than similar medications prescribed by the doctor. It is easy for family members to become emotionally dependent on such pills, and their use should be discouraged except under a doctor's instruction.

GIVING MEDICINES IN THE HOME

When a doctor writes a prescription, it is almost impossible for a layman to read it because of the abbreviations used. If you want to know what is on the prescription form, ask him. This will allow you to check on the pharmacist to be sure he has given you the correct information on the label. The pharmacist gives the prescription and the bottle an RX number so that when you return, he can check to see whether the prescription can be refilled. The numbering system is individual to each pharmacy, and you must return to him in order to get a refill. Most states now require the pharmacist to put the name of the medication on the bottle and in some instances the expiration date also. The label includes all the instructions suggested by the doctor on the prescription blank.

When giving medicine to the patient, remember the five RIGHTS:

- *RIGHT medicine.* The best way to guarantee that family members will take the right medicine is to teach them to read the label—preferably more than once. Many of us reach into the cupboard, take out a bottle, remove one or two pills, and swallow them without ever looking at the label. We just *know* that a certain medicine is on that shelf. But suppose someone has switched things around? This practice can be unsafe, ineffective, uneconomical, and uncomfortable. READ the label and teach family members to do the same.

- *RIGHT patient.* This is a problem only when several family members are on different medications. It is a much greater problem for nurses in the hospital. If you are a patient and the nurse hands you new medications that look unfamiliar, you may wish to say, "Oh, has the doctor changed my medications?" If she has handed you another patient's medications, this will jog her attention and prevent your taking something in error.
- *RIGHT amount.* Follow the instructions on the label. Don't arbitrarily increase the amount because you think you need more than the doctor prescribed. Check with him first.
- *RIGHT time.* Many medications work by building a certain body level of concentration which must be maintained to make the medicine effective. If the label says "every six hours," get up at night and give the patient the medicine. Fortunately, many medications now come in long-acting forms that can be given at less frequent intervals. FOLLOW THE DIRECTIONS.
- *RIGHT manner.* Many medications require special instructions. Instructions may read, "Do not take with food; do not take with liquids. Hold under tongue to dissolve." These instructions increase the effectiveness of the medication and should be followed. If no special instructions are included, the patient may wish to take the pill with milk or follow it with a cracker, either to cover the taste or to eliminate stomach discomfort caused by some medications.

Most small children tend to resist taking medicine. Use a positive, firm, calm approach with no indication by word or manner that you have any doubt that the child will take it. He should not be bribed to take the medicine, and you should be truthful if he asks, "Will it taste bad?" or "Is that all?" He should be praised for his cooperation.

If the child has difficulty swallowing pills, crush them between the bowls of two spoons and add a little fruit puree to the spoon containing the medicine. This works better than dissolving pills in water, since it puts the medicine into suspension and helps cover the bitterness. Don't put the crushed pills into a bowl of cereal or a bottle of milk; you cannot tell how much medicine the child gets if he does not take all of the food. Liquid medications can be given to a baby easily by using a dropper to place the medicine on the baby's tongue.

CARE OF MEDICINE IN THE HOME
Observe the following rules:
- Have a safe place for keeping medicines—a place out of reach of children. Dangerous medicines may be kept in a separate, locked cupboard.
- All medications should be clearly labeled. Have a good light nearby.
- Avoid having solutions that are nonedible (alcohol, kerosene, soap, poisons) in containers from which family members eat or drink (pop bottles, dishes, paper cups).
- Keep the doctor's name and telephone number in a convenient place near the telephone, along with the telephone number for the hospital emergency room and the nearest poison control center. Be sure all family members know where the first-aid book is kept.
- Give medicines only to the one for whom they are prescribed. Medicines are not meant to be shared.
- Encourage family members who have memory problems to make a chart and write down the time at which they take their medicine.
- Chart medicines given the patient on the daily record and note any change in the patient's condition after the medicine has been given.

KEEPING PRESCRIPTION MEDICINES
All medications should have an expiration date on them, since some medicines get weaker and some get stronger with age. Antibiotics, insulin, and vitamin tablets get weaker. Nose drops and tincture of iodine get stronger. Check with the pharmacist to determine how long a medication is useable. Most tablets remain good for several years, but ointments and liquids may be relatively unstable. Check with the doctor before reusing a prescription drug

for a condition that recurs. He may wish to prescribe a different drug.

Dispose of old or unwanted medications safely. Flush them down the toilet or the food disposal. Burying them or putting them in the garbage may allow a pet or a child to find them.

TREATMENTS USING HEAT

Heat applied to an area of the body dilates the blood vessels and increases circulation to the area. Thus heat is used to fight infection, promote healing, relieve pain, relax muscles, and provide warmth. Moist heat is more penetrating than dry heat and can cause burns quickly.

Moist heat includes moist hot packs, a hot bath, steam, or a pan of hot water. The latter is often used for minor infections on the hands or feet. Soaking an infection in hot water for twenty minutes three or four times a day may be all that is necessary to localize it.

Dry heat includes heating pads, sun lamps, and hot water bottles. A hot water bottle can be used as moist heat by wrapping the infected area with a towel wrung out of hot water, placing a piece of plastic around the towel, and laying a hot water bottle on top of the plastic.

The home nurse is responsible for inspection of all heat treatments to make sure the patient is not burned. She should be especially careful if the patient is unconscious, paralyzed, very old, very young, or has any kind of illness or skin condition that would make him especially sensitive to heat.

A hot water bottle is often used by the home nurse to supply either dry or moist heat. The procedure for its use is as follows:

- Test the water. It should be about 120° to 125° or hot enough to be momentarily bearable to your clenched fist.
- Fill the bag 1/2 to 2/3 full. This allows the bag to be more flexible than when completely full.
- Lay the bag flat on the table, holding the neck upright, and allow the air to be expelled. When the water is high in the neck of the bag, the air has all been removed.
- Put the stopper in tightly and hold the bag upside down to check for leaks.
- Dry the bag and place it in a cover. One can be improvised by using a large bath towel. Place the bag at the top edge of the

towel and fold the towel in thirds over it. Proceed as with the bath mitt by bringing the towel up over the top of the bag and tucking it in behind the neck of the bag. A pillow case also makes a good cover for a hot water bottle.

- Change the water about every hour during the procedure.
- When the treatment is finished, empty the bag, hang it upside down to dry, and store it inflated with air and with the stopper in place.

A hot water bottle may be improvised by using a cloth bag of sand, cornmeal, or similar substance, or by using a brick or rock, any of these heated in the oven.

When cold is applied to an area, it reduces the circulation by constricting the capillaries. It is used to reduce swelling, stop bleeding, reduce body temperature, or provide comfort. Ice bags are handled much like hot water bottles. In fact, you can buy a hot water bottle with a wide neck that can be used for ice cubes as well as for hot water. Ice packs can be improvised quickly by wrapping a couple of ice cubes in a washcloth. These are frequently applied to "goose eggs" to help prevent additional swelling and pain. Cold is applied to sprains during the first few hours, but later heat will help the healing process (see first aid for sprains). Cold is also used immediately after a tonsillectomy or a tooth extraction. A rubber kitchen glove placed in the freezer after knots have been made in the fingers, the palm filled with water, and a knot made in the wrist serves admirably as a small ice pack to be held against the cheek after a tooth extraction. Small, heavy, plastic bags with ice cubes in them also work well.

SUMMARY

Medications and treatments can be helpful or dangerous depending on how they are used. As family members become old enough to understand, they should be taught the principles as well as the skills involved in the use of medications and treatments.

THE AGED PATIENT

THE AGING PROCESS

Aging is a continuous process that begins at birth and continues until death. Our bodies are like machines that have the ability to repair themselves but which gradually come to a stop.

Generally speaking, the early adult years are the period of greatest physical activity, and early and middle adulthood are usually the times of establishing a career and rearing a family. Thus, by the time most adults have achieved their personal goals, they are facing their later years. Present-day research indicates that aging does not change one's basic personality or lifestyle. It does, however, bring about a slowing down of most body systems.

Most older people have great assets. Some are emotionally strong, while others have great physical strength. Many retain great intellectual power. Some seem almost immune to illness. Unfortunately, some older people seem unable to adjust to stress, either physical or emotional. They develop a great variety of ailments, each of which may require special attention or help from physicians or family members. If this care is given, most older people can continue to lead happy and useful lives.

Circulatory and Respiratory Systems

Perhaps the most important changes in the body are the cardiovascular changes that occur with aging. Although heart size and rate usually remain about the same as in younger people, it takes the heartbeat a longer period of time to normalize. Thus, after excitement, exercise, or a fall, it takes longer (possibly several hours) for the pulse rate to return to normal.

Narrowing of the blood vessels may obstruct the flow of blood, resulting in such serious forms of illness as heart attacks, strokes, and long-term heart disease. As the blood vessels become less elastic, the heart is forced to work harder to supply blood to the organs. A less serious but annoying problem is a greater sensitivity to cold caused by the slowing of circulation. Poor circulation also causes burns to occur more easily.

The respiratory system also suffers as a consequence of aging. Lung functions are impaired, and the ability to cough is reduced; this increases the danger of respiratory complications such as pneumonia.

The older person may take the following steps in order to decrease these changes in circulation and respiration:

- Keep as active as possible to promote circulation.
- Receive adequate nutrition, maintain a normal body weight, and observe a regular program of exercise.
- Keep the skin dry.
- If open skin lesions occur, obtain medical care.
- Prevent loss of body heat with additional warm clothing.
- Keep floors and house comfortably warm.
- Test bath water before it is used to avoid burns.
- Use rocking chairs and footrests to aid circulation and relax muscles. When lying down, elevate the legs and feet to heart level.
- Stop (or at least cut down on) smoking.

The Nervous System and the Senses

As the aging process continues, sensory and motor impulses and reactions to external stimuli are retarded, causing the person to be slower to react. Not only does this cause a partial loss of communication with the outside world, but it may cause the person to be slower to react to danger.

Modern medicine and science have produced artificial aids that may assist people to overcome some of their sensory loss. If a condition cannot be improved, then others must help the person compensate.

Touch, taste, smell

All these sensory abilities tend to become less acute as a person ages; so far they are usually not correctable. Others may help the older person by taking the following steps:

- Eliminate accident hazards.
- Check for dangers periodically. Dangers such as leaking gas may be easily detected by someone with more acute senses.
- Use caution when applying heat or cold to the older person's body.
- Regard pain as a danger signal.
- Obtain prompt medical care and treatment as needed.

Hearing

Gradual loss may occur in one or both ears. This often happens without the person's being aware of it. Or, if he is aware, he may refuse to acknowledge the fact; he may simply withdraw from group activities rather than admit his problem. In addition to this loss of association, he may become involved in accidents due to his inability to hear.

The hard-of-hearing may be helped in a variety of ways:

- His hearing should be checked in annual physical examinations. Ear infections should get careful attention.
- A hearing aid may be prescribed by a competent specialist and a physician.
- Appropriate surgery for deafness is quite safe and can often be helpful.
- Family members should include him in conversations.
- Speak slowly, distinctly, and without shouting.

Sight

The lens and blood vessels of the eyes may change, resulting in impaired vision. Cataracts and glaucoma may develop. Blurred or restricted vision increases the possibility of accidents. Family members can aid the older person to make the most of his sight by urging him to do the following:

- Have regular eye examinations.
- Seek prompt medical attention for foreign particles in the eye, eye injuries, or inflammation.
- Rest the eyes frequently, especially when doing close work.
- Obtain and use good glasses as prescribed by a doctor.
- Have good light when reading or working.
- Protect eyes against bright sunlight.
- Wear protective goggles or a face shield when working around dangerous tools or equipment.
- Avoid areas which are cluttered or contain hazardous objects.
- Eat an adequate diet. Good health in general is important, for many conditions (such as diabetes) can cause impairments in vision.

Teeth

It should be stressed that teeth can remain in good repair for a lifetime if given proper care; however, teeth are too often neglected. As a result, deterioration starts earlier than is necessary.

Since lost dental enamel is not replaced, there is a tendency toward deterioration of the teeth. The gums also start to change. These changes may cause the loss of teeth or foster infections. Lost teeth may result in facial changes.

Older people should be encouraged to do the following:

- Brush teeth or dentures regularly.
- Obtain dental care regularly.
- Receive prompt attention for diseases of the gums or infections in the mouth.
- Have dentist investigate broken or ragged teeth.
- Refuse to accept extractions instead of possible dental repairs.
- If dentures are needed, make sure they fit well.
- Eat a well balanced diet.

Bones

As the mineral content of the bones changes, the bones become more brittle and are more easily broken. The dangers of breakage are reduced when family members help an aged person in the following ways:

- See that he obtains periodic examinations.
- Help him avoid tripping and falling.
- See that he wears shoes that are well-constructed and have a medium-high heel.
- Equip stairways, ramps, and steps with handrails. Keep them well lighted, uncluttered, and in good repair.
- Make sure rugs are not loose; rugs often are the cause of a fall.
- Keep ice and snow off steps and walkways.

The Feet

Neglect of the feet, though not usually considered serious, can cause the sufferer to become homebound. The elderly are especially susceptible to foot infections because of poorer circulation. The likelihood of problems is made greater by the use of improper footwear.

Most problems an elderly person might have with his feet can be avoided if family members help him observe a few guidelines:

- Keep the feet clean, dry, and free from infections.
- Do not use tight garters.
- Keep the feet warm. Frostbite and gangrene can occur more easily in older persons.

- Wear only shoes that fit well and have proper arch supports.
- Seek prompt medical attention for any symptoms out of the ordinary. Swelling, discoloration of toes, or numbness could indicate a serious condition.
- Avoid scratching or cutting feet and legs, since these heal poorly.
- Soak thick or brittle toenails in water before trimming.
- Do not trim corns or calluses with a knife or razor blade.
- Do not self-treat corns, calluses, ingrown toenails, or other foot conditions.

Skin and Hair

Skin changes may occur as a result of circulatory changes. Thus the skin is drier, bruises occur more easily, and wounds or sores (especially on the legs or feet) are often slow to heal. Decreased glandular activity may cause the hair to become gray, dry, and thin.

A side effect of the bodily changes is that extremities may be swollen, cold, burning, or otherwise uncomfortable.

Help the older person avoid problems with hair and skin by remembering the following precautions:

- Lubricate the skin with mild cream or lotion.
- Use lotion, not alcohol, when giving backrubs.
- Bathe less often and use less soap.
- Use caution when applying external heat because of danger of burning.
- Keep hair clean and brush it well to stimulate scalp circulation.
- Keep extremities clean and dry; elevate them when resting.
- Report any rash or open sore to the doctor.

Elimination

Elimination often raises problems for the aged. Men and women both may find it necessary to urinate frequently. Men may have difficulty urinating because of enlargement of the prostate gland and should check with a doctor to determine whether surgery is necessary. Older people also become constipated easily. Try the following suggestions to help:

- See that he gets an adequate diet, including roughage and plenty of liquids.
- Help him develop regular toilet habits.

- Improvise a bedside toilet for a bedridden patient who can be out of bed for a brief time. Otherwise, leave a bedpan or urinal nearby.

Confinement Problems

Confinement in bed can lead to many other problems if the older patient is not moved frequently. Fluid may collect in his lungs, resulting in a form of pneumonia. Bedsores may occur because of the lessened ability of the skin to tolerate pressure. Muscle tone is readily lost, and extreme weakness may result.

There are two things the family can do to help avoid these conditions:

- Encourage him to be out of bed as much as possible in the home, even though he may find it simpler to remain in bed.
- If he is bedfast, the family should work with a doctor or physical therapist to determine the best exercise program for him.

Medication and Immunizations

Drugs

Drugs are one of the major health aids available to the sick, and they offer to the aging hope of maintaining good health longer than ever before. Still, if drugs are misused, they can bring disastrous results. As a person ages, a problem occurs that is not generally found in younger people: since medications are excreted more slowly from an older person's body, there is danger of an accumulation of drugs, resulting in mental confusion. If improperly taken, drugs can even cause death.

These undesirable effects can be avoided if an elderly person is aware of these precautions:

- Ask questions of the doctor until instructions for use are clear.
- Do not self-diagnose or self-doctor.
- Take only medicine prescribed by a doctor—do not try the prescriptions of friends or family.
- Inform the doctor of previous problems with drugs and tell him what drugs are currently being taken.
- Discontinue use immediately of any drug causing nausea, vomiting, hives, skin rashes, inflammation of the eyes, exhaustion, or confusion. See physician immediately.

- Label all medicine bottles in large, clear letters. Discard old medicines regularly.
- Important: carry in wallet or purse information about drugs or special treatments needed; also have the name and telephone number of the doctor.

Immunizations

Infectious diseases are generally much harder on older people than on younger ones. For this reason, the aged need to receive proper immunization against diseases that threaten them. Since some people already are immune to certain diseases, while others have lost immunity to some diseases, each person should consult with his doctor about what immunizations are necessary.

Many retirees engage in foreign travel; therefore they will need certain immunizations. It is best if these are started early to reduce the possibility of ill effects. These effects are more pronounced with the aged than with other groups.

Check with a physician for specific immunizations that should be received, but the following are usually given special attention in the aged:

- Smallpox—if traveling in certain countries.
- Diphtheria
- Tetanus (This has a high mortality rate for those over 40.)
- Poliomyelitis
- Influenza (Flu hits the aged harder than other groups. Try to get an immunization annually, before epidemics begin.)
- Gamma Globulin, if recommended for the specific area

Nutrition and Eating

As a person ages and his activity decreases, he requires less food. Consequently, many older people tend to put on excess weight. On the other hand, the taste buds become less sensitive, and some people become indifferent to food; these people may find eating to be too much trouble, and malnutrition may result.

Many complaints of the aged concerning general weakness, irritability, or some psychological symptoms may be due to malnutrition. The source of such malnutrition is principally inadequate intake of protein, calcium, and vitamins.

A few suggestions for the aged to maintain adequate nutrition may be helpful:

- Adjust meal size and frequency. Small, frequent meals may be better than two or three large meals a day.
- Reduce caloric intake to a level consistent with physical activity. Try to maintain the weight recommended for height and age.
- Fasting or drastic diet is not desirable as a means to lose weight.
- Eat a balanced diet. This should generally be low fat, medium carbohydrate, and high protein.
- An adequate supply of fruit, vegetables, and milk will provide the necessary vitamins and minerals.
- If an adequate and balanced diet is maintained, vitamin pills (usually expensive) will not be necessary.
- Heavy meals should be avoided at all times, but especially before going to bed.
- Unless otherwise advised by a doctor, salt intake should be increased during hot, humid weather, and daily fluid intake should be increased to six or eight glasses.
- Avoid the habitual use of laxatives; eat fruits, vegetables, and other foods with bulk to prevent constipation.
- Avoid foods that have been hard to digest in the past. Usually, these would be fried, highly seasoned, high in fat foods and gravies, heavy sauces, and foods heavy in carbohydrates.
- If a sudden and persistent loss of appetite occurs, get medical attention.

Sex and Aging

As a person ages, the sex organs change, causing a loss of the capacity for reproduction; the needs or desires for sex, however, change much more slowly. All these changes are gradual, and well-adjusted persons do not have sexual problems because of aging.

A recent study has shown that 80 to 85 percent of married couples between sixty and sixty-five engage in sexual intercourse. Seventy percent of those between sixty-five and seventy do also. Potency is retained by some 50 percent of men after age seventy, and there is little loss of sexual desire by women after menopause. Even the loss of the uterus and ovaries has little influence on sexual desires and capabilities. Thus, *elderly people should not consider sexual activity in any way abnormal or inappropriate.*

It is normal for some concern to be felt by women from forty-five to fifty-five who go through menopause. This means an end to their child-bearing years, and some women become worried and depressed. Just as with pregnancy, the changing hormonal adjustment within the body may produce annoying symptoms such as hot flashes, irritability, excess perspiration, headaches, or dizziness. At the same time, the monthly menstrual cycles tend to become irregular and to decrease in duration and amount. The symptoms vary tremendously from woman to woman; many women have no problems during menopause. Regular medical examinations including a pap smear should be obtained throughout this period.

Physical Activity and Exercise

Regulated physical activity is absolutely necessary if an older person hopes to maintain his strength. Exercise maintains the power of the heart and the lungs, and preserves general muscle tone.

Nevertheless, he should use caution in exercising. He should be aware of the following ideas in regulating his exercise:

- Avoid competitive athletics.
- Concentrate on exercise that does not involve sudden strenuous efforts. Cycling, walking, and swimming are good.
- Exercise regularly, not just on weekends or during summers.
- Avoid exercise under such adverse conditions as extremes in temperature, the period following a heavy meal, or the times when he is not feeling completely well.
- He should never push an activity to the point of discomfort or distress.
- He should try to find relaxing activities.

Sleep

The amount of sleep needed varies greatly from individual to individual. However, certain trends are common among the elderly: insomnia, sleeping shorter periods at night, and napping during the day.

Here are a few guidelines for you to suggest to the older person:

- Generally, he should get enough sleep to awaken refreshed.
- He should consult a physician for diagnosis and treatment of the causes of insomina.
- He should not rely on sleeping tablets.
- He should keep active during the day, but should not become overtired or exceed the limits of tolerance.

Accident Prevention

The greatest hazard to the aged who are in good health is accidents: it is the third greatest cause of death among older men and fifth among older women. In addition, every fatal accident is probably matched by 200 nonfatal but disabling ones.

The risk of accidents is increased by impaired vision, hearing, taste, smell, and reflexes. Older people should be made aware of their own limitations and taught to compensate for them. Driving may become dangerous as one's senses become less alert. The age at which this occurs varies considerably.

HOUSING

As a person ages, his body loses some of its abilities. Proper housing can help minimize these losses and protect the individual. Some suggestions that might be of value include the following:

- The house should protect the individual from extreme heat, extreme cold, extreme dampness, and overexposure to sun, heavy winds, or any other extremes of weather.
- It should take into account any special needs to meet limitations of the individual such as orthopedic or cardiac conditions.
- Living quarters should have easy access to toilet and kitchen and require minimal use of stairs.
- Floors should be nonslip materials, especially in bathrooms; there should be no loose rugs.
- Bathtubs and showers should have grab bars and non-slip bottoms.
- Closets and cabinets should not require stools or frequent bending.
- Fireguards should be provided for fireplaces, stoves, and radiators.
- Labor-saving devices should be available as necessary.
- Either electric stoves or vents to the outside for oil or gas stoves should be provided.
- The elderly person should have a telephone and a buzzer in his quarters to summon help in case of emergency.

CLOTHING

Since clothing plays an important role in both physical and mental health, the elderly should be encouraged to consider both functional and aesthetic values in choosing clothes. They should consider cost, fit, and style. In addition, the following points may prove useful in selecting proper clothing:

- Dress should take into account changes in season and weather.
- Clothing should be easy to put on and take off, particularly when the individual has some disability.
- Choose nice-looking, comfortable clothes; avoid tight garments, garters, and belts.
- Shoes should look good and fit well, should be comfortable, and should provide support for walking. Slip-on shoes eliminate the necessity for stooping to tie them.
- Foundation garments can improve appearance by supporting sagging muscles, but avoid tight corsets and girdles that might interfere with breathing.

PSYCHOLOGICAL CONSIDERATIONS

General

People everywhere, of all ages, want about the same things from life: health, security, something worthwhile to do, someone to love, and a place to live where they can feel comfortable. Older people are often faced with failing health, insecurity, and failing productivity. If, in addition, they feel they are not wanted, needed, or noticed, they may face more stress than they can stand.

Family members can help older people by following a few basic guidelines:

- Show respect for their experience. Seek their opinions.
- Involve them in appropriate activities.
- Do not take offense at their disposition and personality changes; understand their problems instead.
- Do not hurry them. Impatience and doing for them are threats to their dignity and may cause a loss of a feeling of independence.
- Do not criticize them or complain about them.
- Always keep the lines of communication open.
- Remind them that they are only as old as they feel and think.
- Love them.
- When helping them, remember to:
  - Make all instructions clear and concise.
  - Break tasks down and demonstrate them if necessary.
  - Allow adequate time for them to perform tasks.

- Speak clearly but don't shout unless hearing is severly impaired.
- Encourage the patients to feed themselves and give themselves medicine even though it takes longer.

Hospitalization

When hospitalized, the older person often seems completely confused, even if he normally has no problem caring for himself. He may lose track of time, become disoriented as to time and place, or become forgetful.

The following suggestions may help:
- Take along to the hospital some of his personal possessions.
- Have family members spend time with him.
- Help him understand hospital routine and orient him to the physical layout of the area.
- Give him a clock with large numbers and a calendar so that he will not lose track of time.
- Provide verbal clues and involve the patient in everyday activities around him to help combat forgetfulness.

Personal Hygiene

As a person becomes more dependent physically, he may develop poor hygiene habits and may show less interest in clothes and personal appearance. Neglect of these regular habits is often a symptom of depression and withdrawal; if such is the case, the conditions causing the neglect must be treated as well as the neglect itself. The neglect can often be curtailed by encouragement and assistance from family members. The home nurse should always encourage him to do as much as possible for himself, even if it takes much longer, for this will help maintain his dignity and self-respect.

Mental Processes and Memory

Elderly people are often troubled by the slowdown of their mental processes and the realization that they cannot remember things as well as they used to; if friends and family criticize them, they may quit trying. They also worry when they find themselves reminiscing; this, however, can be of value to them, strengthening the ego and giving new meaning to life.

A few suggestions for family members to help the older person with these matters are as follows:

- Give him a notebook in which he can write himself little reminders about where he is to go and what he is to do.
- Seek his opinions and experience.
- Give him a voice in decisions that will affect him whenever possible.
- Do not criticize him if he forgets.
- Help him set up an established routine.
- Provide verbal clues to jog his memory.

Leisure Time

Another problem often facing the elderly is the decline in their productivity. In our work-oriented society, we tend to look down on those who are nonproductive, even ourselves. Since most older people are retired (a condition increasingly accepted by society), they need to develop a positive attitude toward leisure. This can be done by finding satisfying and constructive uses of leisure time. Age does not decrease our ability to learn new things.

To help the aged person adjust to leisure, urge and help him to do the following things:

- Do what he enjoys doing (not what he thinks he should be doing).
- Find new ways to use old skills; develop hobbies.
- Look for opportunities to help others.
- Do nothing at all if that is what he prefers to do.

SUMMARY

Aging can be a period of fulfillment and pleasure when a person is surrounded by those he loves and is physically and mentally healthy. The vast majority of older people live busy, normal lives in their communities. Preparation for a happy old age may be aided by the following suggestions:

- Receive regular physical examinations, dental checkups, and necessary immunizations.
- Eat a balanced diet.
- Keep up a program of regular exercise.
- Receive adequate and restful sleep.
- Avoid harmful habits and excesses.
- Do not self-diagnose or self-treat.

- Learn to enjoy and use leisure time.
- Form and keep healthy relationships both within and without the family.
- Maintain personal hygiene and appearance.
- Accept personal strengths and limitations.
- If active in a church, maintain the affiliation and practices of the church.
- Remember that the best defenses against problems are good health, good humor, and a busy life full of service.

TERMINAL ILLNESS

We all need to remember that life itself is a terminal experience. For a person with a strong religious faith, death is simply one of the necessary steps toward eternal life. For one lacking faith, however, to be told he has a terminal illness is a frightening experience. This chapter is intended to help us understand the process a person goes through in accepting terminal illness. Like the process of grief it is made up of a series of definite steps that most people follow.

FIRST STAGE: DENIAL

Almost without exception, a person who is told he has a terminal illness will react with the statement, "No, not me, it can't be me." Even if he is not told but arrives at the conclusion on his own, he will still deny it. In our sub-conscious minds we somehow believe that we are immortal. Most people, if asked, will indicate that they expect to die suddenly—that they will never actually have to face the idea of death.

This temporary state of shock and denial eventually gives way to partial acceptance, yet at times the patient will suddenly revert to denial. The need to deny comes and goes, and a perceptive listener will attempt to be aware of this without calling the patient's attention to the contradictions. Denial functions as a buffer against something too frightening to accept. A stronger, better adjusted individual can deal with the reality better and appears less frightened. He may wish to talk to family members about his feelings as well as his desire to accomplish certain things before death occurs. As family members we often attempt to postpone such conversations because of our own fears, but in doing so, we do the patient a real disservice. Instead, we should be willing listeners when he is ready to talk. He needs most of all someone he can trust, who is nonjudgmental and completely accepting when he opens up and shares his feelings of loneliness.

SECOND STAGE: ANGER

When the first stage of denial gives way, it is replaced by anger, rage, envy, and resentment. The patient rants, "Why me, of all people?" This is a difficult stage for the family, since the anger is often projected toward those around him. The doctors are no good, the family doesn't care, the diet is terrible, the restrictions are insane; everywhere the patient looks he finds grievances. If the family fails to realize where the anger is coming from, they may throw up their hands in despair. They don't realize that the patient is proclaiming loudly, "I'm alive. I want attention. I'm not dead yet." The danger is that family members will take his anger personally and will respond with anger. They begin to avoid the patient or shorten their visits. Visitors from outside the family may find themselves in the same category.

A patient who is loved, respected, and understood, who is given time to vent his anger without anger in return will soon lower his voice and reduce his demands. Family members in turn will realize that expressing anger, even though it is irrational, may give the patient great relief and help him along in his task of adjustment. Accepting anger is not an easy thing to do. It takes family members who are not defensive and afraid, who can honestly let the patient know that he is a valuable human being who will be allowed to function as long as he can.

THIRD STAGE: BARGAINING

The stage of bargaining varies from patient to patient, is less well known by psychologists, and tends to appear and disappear. Most of us use bargaining in various life experiences to get what we want, and every patient knows that it is a tool that may help. Most bargaining is really an attempt to postpone the inevitable.

Most bargains are made with God and are often kept secret so that family members are not aware of promises made. If a patient does choose to talk about them, family members should not brush the promises aside but should listen and help where possible. A common bargain is one in which the patient promises the Lord that he will live righteously if he is allowed to live a little longer. These promises help the patient to make peace with his maker and often give him great comfort.

FOURTH STAGE: DEPRESSION

When the patient can no longer deny his illness, his anger and rage usually give way to a sense of great loss. He becomes weaker, begins to have more symptoms, and smiles less often.

Our initial reaction to sad people is to try to cheer them up. We try to help them see the bright side of life. This may help if the patient is feeling guilty about the things he should be doing, since it reassures him. But if the depression is the type which is a preparation for acceptance, the patient does not want to be cheered. Rather he wishes to express his sorrow so that the acceptance will be easier, and he will be grateful to those who will listen without constantly being cheerful. This may be a time of withdrawal. The patient may express a desire not to have too many visitors who distract him from his task of preparation. Again the family needs to sense the patient's mood, realizing that it may change from day to day or from hour to hour.

FIFTH STAGE: ACCEPTANCE

If the patient has had enough time to work through the first four stages, he will finally reach the stage where he is neither angry nor depressed. He seems at peace and sleeps undisturbed for increasing periods of time. It is not a happy time, but it is as though the struggle is over and he awaits the final journey. This may be a time when the family needs more support than the patient. They seem unable to understand the patient's need to be left alone, his lack of interest in the outside world, his uncommunicative moods. He seems content if family members sit in silence, yet he needs the assurance that they are there. A squeeze of the hand may be as meaningful as an infinite number of words.

There are a few patients who continue to fight to the end, expressing hope and fighting acceptance, and if a patient chooses this approach, a wise family will support him and not insist that he be accepting. In fact, all patients, even those who become most accepting seem to leave open the possibility that something will happen to save them. It is often this hope that sustains them through the weeks and months. Family members should not become hopeless themselves; yet they need to accept the patient's sense of readiness for death.

In a sense, family members face the same stages of acceptance as does the patient. They need to share their emotions with each other as well as with the patient. It is unfortunate that people feel unable to talk about death among themselves or with patients. If they could do this, they would be less frightened. So often they hesitate because of their own sense of inadequacy. They end up using a forced cheerfulness that may completely alienate the patient. Instead, they should follow the patient's lead.

DEATH AND CONSOLING

When death occurs in our own family or when we wish to console others who have suffered the loss of a loved one, we should remember that the grief process is a long one and varies tremendously from person to person. The most meaningful help we can give any person—child or adult—is to share his feelings and allow him to work them out, whether the feelings are rational or irrational. Such help can often shorten the grief period and facilitate the person's adjustment to the loss.

HOME SAFETY HINTS

"Mommie, Mommie," cries a voice high-pitched with pain and terror, "Hurry! I just fell down the stairs and hurt my knee and it's bleeding something awful." How often have you heard a similar cry in your home? Things like this may not happen every day, but they occur often enough to make all of us aware of the importance of home safety. Approximately seventeen million children are injured some time or another during their childhood. Each year a total of 50,000 children are crippled and almost two million are temporarily incapacitated by accidental injury. One child out of every three is injured severely enough each year in the United States to require medical attention. . . . During any one year, the statisticians tell us, "5,500 accidental deaths in children under five years of age occur in the home." (Vincent J. Fonlara, M.D. *A Parent's Guide to Child Safety,* [New York: Thomas Y. Crowell Co., 1973], p. xx, Preface).

Sociologists, psychologists, and religious leaders plead with us to make the family unit the basis of our lives—to spend more time together working and playing. If, then, the home is to be the center of our activities, how can we make it a safe place to be?

There are many answers to the above question, but let's approach the problem by asking some additional questions.

- How well organized is your home? Do you have a place for things, and are they kept there when not in use? Perhaps a do-it-yourself handyman or older son could help build a storage spot for special equipment, or how about tackling such a project yourself? Many books and magazines give step-by-step instructions for building storage areas. Go ahead. Try it.

- What about poisonous substances? Are they clearly labeled and out of reach of small children? Don't forget grandchildren or friendly neighborhood children who may frequent your home. Every year 600,000 children eat potentially poisonous substances of various kinds. Of these, some 500 children die a year. Aspirin, insecticides, kerosene, detergents, bleaches, and polishes are common causes of death by poisoning. The following are rules each family should observe:

- Never store nonedible substances in containers used for eating, i.e., rubbing alcohol in a cup; gasoline or cleaning fluid in a pop bottle; pills in a cereal bowl. If you store water in bleach bottles, be sure family members know which bottles contain water and which contain bleach.
- Keep medicine out of reach of children but in an area where the light is good. Be sure bottles are clearly labeled and family members make a practice of reading the label before they take any medicine. A couple of vitamin C tablets taken in place of aspirin may be harmless, but they do little to help a headache.
- If you store prescription medicines, use them only as directed by the doctors and be aware of the expiration date. Some drugs get stronger with age, while others weaken.
- Garden products such as pesticides and insecticides may be very dangerous if they are inhaled or absorbed through the skin. Follow the instructions on the label carefully. Taken internally they are deadly; keep them locked up out of the reach of children.
- Household detergents and cleaning materials may be highly caustic. Keep them out of reach. Fifteen percent of all calls to poison control centers throughout the country involve questions about the ingestion of detergents in children under five years of age. Remember, aspirin, detergent, or zinc oxide may be as tantalizing to them as ice cream is to you.

- Are you a collector? Many of us are, and we keep assuring ourselves that we'll find uses for those old refrigerators, cars, bottles, rags, papers, or cans. Remember that such things as an old refrigerator, a freezer, or a car may be a death trap for a child. And rags and papers stored near heating equipment may start a fire that will snuff out the lives of loved ones.
- Had you considered that falls are a common cause of injury among all age groups but particularly among older members of the family who are less agile or whose vision is impaired? Keep stairways lighted and uncluttered, toys picked up, and rugs anchored. Outside the home, be sure that snow and ice are promptly removed as these may be the cause of serious falls.
People also fall from high places—porches, balconies, windows, ladders, and trees—as well as on slippery surfaces such as bathtubs, highly polished floors, or wet linoleum.

- How dangerous is your kitchen area? Are there hazards which you have learned from experience to avoid? Remember that younger family members can benefit from your experience in working with stoves, knives, and hot utensils. Keep pressurized containers away from excessive heat that may cause them to explode. Be careful when cutting the lids from cans. Watch for loose clothing when working over the stove. Wipe up spills from the floor. Beware of glass or sharp metal in reaching into the waste containers to retrieve something. Never stick a fork or knife into a plugged-in toaster to retrieve bread. Don't store the cookie jar on a high shelf where a child must climb to reach it. Don't leave cords dangling for toddlers to jerk. Keep handles of pots and pans turned out of reach of children. The smell of gas is a danger signal; don't light a match to find the source of the gas leak. An explosion may result. If you use gas appliances, follow the instructions and have them inspected by a qualified workman when necessary.

- What about safety in the bathroom? Do family members know that electricity and water don't mix and that they should never touch electrically operated appliances if their bodies or hands are wet? Hands should be dry when operating electrical tools, switches, or appliances.

Unfortunately, there is no way to make a home completely safe, since many complex factors enter in. Although some accidents are due to lack of knowledge, especially among children, the majority occur to individuals who knew the safety hazards and ignore them. Psychological factors such as fear, anger, nervousness, or anxiety often have a strong influence on our behavior. During such periods we tend to be less alert and less attentive to what we are doing.

Home safety must become a family affair. Have an evening's project in which the whole family checks the house for areas of danger. Assign various family members to remedy defects in their area of responsibility. Even little ones can help eliminate dangerous clutter from toys scattered about. Have a family plan for emergencies such as a fire. Have the scouts in your family teach all of you basic first-aid principles. Have the necessary phone numbers, such as doctor, hospital, fire department, and poison control center listed near the telephone. Practice role-playing some emergencies. Even a three-year-old can save a life by dialing "0."

Encourage older family members to be constantly aware of what your family members are doing. It may take all of you to prevent the baby from choking on a button or the three-year-old from playing with matches. Make home safety something that all family members are constantly involved in. It is more than just Mother's responsibility. Children don't like to be constantly scolded, but many teaching opportunities present themselves when minor accidents do occur. Other family members can learn from each experience, and thus the whole family can grow in their knowledge of safety. Sometimes we are tempted to prevent children from using tools and equipment that may be dangerous, but a better approach is to take the time to teach them how to use available equipment wisely. A little time spent in this area may avert a tragedy. The following information is taken from *Relief Society Courses of Study,* 1974.

SAFETY CHECKLISTS

General Home Safety:
- Are all old newspapers and other flammable materials removed promptly from the basement or storage area?
- Are electric cords that are exposed to water coated with rubber?
- Are nonflammable cleaning fluids used and then only out-of-doors?
- Is an inspection made once a month to check for any special hazards?
- Are garage doors left open while the car motor is running?
- Are snow and slush promptly removed from porch and walks?
- Do you store sharp or pointed kitchen utensils away from the reach of children and make sure they cannot upset hot foods or come in contact with flames or burners on the stove?
- Are small objects that could be swallowed kept away from babies and small children?
- Are obstacles such as toys, chairs, and other objects kept out of the traffic areas of the home?
- Is the bath area safe from conditions that might cause falls or other accidents?
- Are the electrical wiring and fuses or breakers in good repair and adequate for current needs?

- Do all family members know what to do in case of accident or emergency?
- Has the family had instruction concerning action in case of fire in the home, held fire drills, and practiced other safety measures?
- Have you done everything in your power to make your home safe and your family safety conscious?
- Is ice on the doorstep and walks covered with sand or other gritty material?
- Are porch steps and walks unobstructed?
- Do porch steps have a strong handrail?
- Are emergency telephone numbers posted, and do all family members know how to obtain help in an emergency?

Kitchen:
- Is the floor clean and free from hazards such as upturned linoleum edges?
- Are electric appliances disconnected from the outlet when not in use?
- Is the electric iron rested on a proper stand when not in use?
- Are the handles of pots and pans on the stove turned out of the reach of children?
- Are receptacles with water emptied immediately after using?
- Are all gas connections checked twice a year to detect leaks or defects?
- Are knives and other sharp instruments kept out of the reach of children?
- Do all family members know that in using a knife they must always cut away from the body?

Other Rooms:
- Are small rugs anchored so that they do not slip on polished floors?
- Are the edges of rugs prevented from curling?
- Is there a storage place for toys, and are they kept there when not in use?
- Is nonskid wax used on floors?
- Are scissors kept out of the reach of small children?
- Are extension cords placed where they will not be tripped over?
- Are stairs well lighted and unobstructed?
- Is carpeting in good repair and fastened securely to the floor?
- Are there secure gates at the bottoms and tops of stairs to

protect young children?

- Is a rubber mat placed in the tub?
- Are medicines and poisonous substances placed in a locked cabinet or other place inaccessible to children?
- Are all poisons kept in clearly marked containers, and are labels double checked before using?
- Are little children never left alone in the bathroom?
- Is the passageway from the bed to the door unobstructed?
- Are window screens securely installed?
- Are drawers and cupboards always closed when not in use?
- Is there a convenient light switch for emergency night use?
- Are safeguards provided to prevent children from falling out of cribs and beds?

Vehicles and Traffic:

- Are all vehicles that are owned or driven maintained in a good state of repair?
- Are seat belts always worn by the driver and by passengers for whom belts have been provided?
- Are children safe in car seats and protected against any hazard in the car? Are they never left alone in a car?
- Do you avoid driving when you are upset, tired, or not in complete control of your emotions and reactions?
- Do you observe all traffic rules and safety precautions when driving?
- Do you drive defensively?
- Do you look both ways before crossing streets, use crosswalks, avoid stepping into the roadway from behind parked cars, and observe other pedestrian cautions?
- Do you lock car doors and raise windows at least part way, restrain children, and take other action to prevent them from falling from or in the car?
- Do you and your family always walk on the sidewalk or facing traffic?
- Do your children avoid playing in the street?
- Do your children observe special caution near traffic going to and coming from school?
- Do you properly control your children when you are using buses or other public transportation?

Safety in the Area of the Home:

- Has your family done all in its power to remedy or encourage neighbors to help in removing or safeguarding any accident hazards in your neighborhood?

- Is there a safe area near home where your children can play?
- Have you taught your children never to play with sharp or pointed objects, never to throw rocks or other objects, and to avoid dangerous places?
- Have you and your family learned how to swim properly and in company with others, and do you take proper precautions around any body of water?
- Is the yard and immediate vicinity of your home free of trash, broken bottles, tin cans, barbed wire, and other potentially dangerous objects?

FIRST AID

PART ONE: GENERAL PRINCIPLES

Most of us, at one time or another, have been faced with caring for a seriously ill or injured person. Sometimes the injury is minor, but often it is serious; we then wish desperately for an expert to tell us what to do.

First aid may be defined as the immediate care given to a person who has been injured or suddenly taken ill. It includes self-help and home care if medical assistance is not available or is delayed. It includes a willingness to care for the victim, to reassure him, and to give him confidence.

Often first aid makes the difference between life and death. Even in less serious situations, it is a great comfort to the victim to feel that someone competent has taken over.

Accidents are a frequent cause of death or disability throughout the world, especially among children. In the USA they are the major cause of death of persons from one to thirty-seven and the fourth leading cause of death for all ages (National Safety Council).

Priorities When an Accident Occurs

Prompt action may save a life, and a first-aider must have some general principles in mind. These five activities must be carried out quickly as the first-aider assesses the situation and others seek help:

- *Unless it is necessary* to rescue the victim from such things as water, fire or gas, *do not move him* until you are certain that moving him will cause no further physical damage. Keep him quiet and comfortable. Do not let him get up and walk around. Enlist the help of bystanders to summon appropriate help, direct traffic, and help with any crowd which gathers.
- See if the victim is breathing. If he is not, be sure the air passage is open and give mouth-to-mouth resuscitation.
- Check pulse at carotid area (the artery in the neck just below

the central part of the jawbone). If it is absent, start cardiac massage *only* if an experienced person is available.

- Control severe bleeding by using direct pressure on the wound.
- Check whether the victim has swallowed harmful chemicals and, if so, give first aid for poisoning.
- Check the pulse, respiration, and color to determine whether the victim is in shock.

Once the extent of the problem is evident, the first-aider can proceed:

- Move the patient as little as possible, especially where back and neck injuries are suspected.
- Check for identification; it may include medical information. Look for special medicines in the victim's possession.
- Check methodically for other injuries.
- Ask questions of the victim if possible, or of others who observed the accident or saw the person collapse, but avoid unnecessary conversation. Respect a person's privacy about anything you may learn.
- Help the victim to maintain normal body temperature. Prevent chilling, but don't just pile blankets or coats on him.
- Loosen tight clothing and, if necessary, rip or cut away clothing to allow for care of injuries. Do not expose the victim unnecessarily.
- Check for stains around the mouth if poisoning is suspected.
- Carry out first aid as needed and remain with the victim until a qualified person such as a physician, an ambulance crew, a rescue squad, or a police officer arrives.

When administering help, a first-aider should remember these limitations:

- Do not feel obligated to explain to bystanders what you are doing. Do not attempt to make a diagnosis.
- Know your limitations. Don't try to do procedures you know nothing about; you may only cause further injury.
- Never give food or water to unconscious patients.
- Never attempt to tell more experienced people what to do.

Legal Implications of First Aid

Let us consider at this point the legal implications of administering first aid. Most first aid is administered within your family circle where legal factors are not a major concern. Outside the family we should offer help when needed. If you act in the best interest of the person in trouble and keep in mind your limitations, you need not worry about being held liable. Basic first aid seeks to give comfort, to prevent the victim from further injury, and to sustain him until medical help arrives. Many places have "Good Samaritan Laws" to protect those who offer emergency first aid to the ill and injured.

Summary

Having a knowledge of first aid serves several purposes. It prepares a person to care for family members or for himself when sudden illness or injury occurs. It makes him more aware of safety measures which will help to prevent accidents. It also prepares him to help others when disaster, either natural or man-made, strikes an area.

PART TWO: EQUIPMENT AND SUPPLIES

First-aid Kits

Since no one has ever been able to create a totally accident-free society, it is essential that each family have the necessary first-aid supplies to take care of emergencies. In general, first-aid supplies should be located in a convenient area with good lighting. They may be kept in the kitchen or bathroom of a home and should be out of reach of small children. They should be kept in a separate container which can easily be moved to the person who is injured. It is useful to keep an extra kit in the car.

Any box may be used as a container for first-aid supplies but should close tightly to keep out dust and moisture. A metal, wood, or plastic container with a hinged cover, such as a small tool chest, tackle box, or surplus ammunition box, will work well. Compartments within the box help to keep supplies organized. Family members should be familiar with the kit so that they can find the things they need quickly. A first-aid booklet should be kept with the kit. It is best not to have the kit locked since precious moments may be lost hunting for the key.

Although it is usually best to check with your doctor for any specific medicines or supplies your family might need on an emergency basis, the following are standard first-aid supplies:

Permanent Equipment

scissors	thermometers (oral and rectal)
tweezers	hot water bottle
knife	ice bag
measuring cup	flashlight
medicine dropper	splints
	sling material

triangular bandages (muslin, sheeting, or other soft material—approximately 40" square, but cut in two diagonally)

rope

wooden splints: 1/2 x 4 x 30; 1/2 x 3 x 14 approximate measurements—subject to materials available)

blanket (stored alongside the kit according to space limits)

Expendable Supplies

soap	safety pins
matches	adhesive tape
batteries for flashlight	constricting band
razor blades	cotton
package of needles	

elastic bandage (If not available, the triangular bandage can be used.)

six rolls of gauze bandage (If not available, the triangular bandage can be used.)

sterile gauze dressings (If not available, sterile dressings can be made by using a hot iron to sterilize a clean handkerchief or piece of cloth—preferably white and preferably cotton. These can be sterilized in advance by thoroughly heating and ironing three cloths and folding one of them inside the other two without touching the inside sterile cloth bandage. This will make a relatively germ-free bandage—at least for awhile. If time permits and facilities are available, or if it has been pre-packaged for a long time, it can be resterilized with an iron again before using.)

package of small dressing with tape

paper bags (to use for hyperventilation)

Medications (Non-prescription)
ipecac syrup (to induce vomiting)
powdered activated charcoal (to absorb swallowed poison)
bicarbonate of soda (baking soda)
ammonia (small bottle of aromatic spirits)
calamine lotion (for sunburn, insect bites, etc.)
rubbing alcohol or other antiseptic

Medications (Prescription—Optional)
diarrhea preparation
antibiotic ointment

Small personal kits are often used by those who hike, hunt, camp or fish and should include bandages, matches (paraffin-treated so they will burn longer and be waterproof), soap and washcloth, sterile pads, adhesive tape, and a triangular bandage.

First-aid kits and supplies should be checked and replenished regularly. Supplies that are old or contaminated are unsafe and should be replaced. Usually it is better to use tubes or plastic bottles to eliminate breakage. All supplies should be well labeled and kept in an organized way.

Most of us at one time or another have to improvise first-aid equipment. Anything placed next to a wound should be sterile if possible. Cloth which is freshly laundered, ironed, placed in an oven at 350°F (177°C) for three hours, boiled for 15 minutes, and then dried, or held and cleaned over the fire is considered sterile. Fluff cotton or open weave material will stick to the wound and will be difficult to remove. In an emergency where bleeding must be stopped, towels, sheets, napkins, a torn blouse or slip, a freshly laundered handkerchief, even ties or socks may be used. Pick the cleanest available material and remember not to touch the surface which will be placed on the wound. Over the dressing an improvised bandage may be applied. Use strips of knit material, material cut on the bias, or nylon stockings. The bandage need not be sterile but should be as clean as possible.

Summary

Every family should have first-aid supplies on hand in case of an emergency and should be acquainted with the contents of the kit. Some practice situations involving emergencies could make family members feel much more secure should a real emergency arise.

PART THREE: ILLNESSES REQUIRING IMMEDIATE ATTENTION

Many times we are faced with sudden illness not caused by accident but which we must assess and care for. One of the most baffling of these situations occurs when a person is unconscious and the first-aider is unable to get any helpful information to indicate the cause. Unconsciousness may be caused by poisoning, lack of oxygen, head injury or severe shock. Each of these conditions will be discussed in a later lesson.

Let us consider some other causes of unconsciousness:

- Fainting is due to a temporary decrease of blood and oxygen supply to the brain. It may occur without warning or may be preceded by paleness, sweating, dizziness, disturbances of vision and nausea. Recovery usually occurs spontaneously, shortly after the victim has been placed in a reclining position. He may be pale and weak afterwards and should be watched carefully and allowed to rest. If spontaneous recovery does not occur in a few minutes, medical help should be obtained.

- Convulsions are a form of unconsciousness accompanied by violent jerking movements and rigidity of the muscles. The person often appears blue about the lips and may drool. In some children convulsions may accompany a high fever; and though they may be frightening, the convulsion itself is not dangerous. Other causes of convulsions may include head injury or severe infections, such as meningitis. Some people have a convulsive disorder known as epilepsy. *The first-aid treatment of convulsions is aimed at preventing the patient from hurting himself.* If he should stop breathing, begin mouth-to-mouth resuscitation. Do *not* place a blunt object between his teeth. Do *not* restrain him, do *not* give him liquids, and do *not* put a child who is convulsing in a tub of water. If the convulsion recurs or lasts for a long period of time, seek medical help.

- A stroke is caused by the spontaneous rupture of a blood vessel in the brain or formation of a clot in a vessel in the brain. These occur most frequently in older people suffering from hardening of the arteries. Unconsciousness, paralysis of one side of the body, unequal size of the pupils, and difficulty in breathing and swallowing often accompany a severe stroke. First be sure the patient is breathing. Then position him on his side. Avoid giving anything by mouth and get medical help as soon as possible.

118

- Occasionally an unconscious patient is a diabetic who has had too little or too much insulin. He may have some type of identification indicating he is diabetic. Unless the person is a member of your family and you are thoroughly familiar with his treatment, it would probably be better to seek medical help rather than to attempt first-aid measures.

Another category of sudden illness occurring at home involves acute pain. Often it is difficult to distinguish between pain, fear, and anxiety. You should be calm and reassuring while asking questions that will help determine the source of the pain.

- One serious form of pain occurs with a heart attack caused by blockage of one of the blood vessels supplying the heart muscle. A severe attack may cause unconsciousness, and the patient may die quickly. In the conscious patient, there may be persistent chest pain in the middle of the front part of the chest, shortness of breath, pallor and perspiration (indicating shock), and extreme prostration (exhaustion). He may be able to breathe better if he is propped up. First aid includes mouth-to-mouth resuscitation if the patient is not breathing and getting an ambulance equipped with oxygen.

- Severe abdominal pain may be due to appendicitis, food poisoning, a hernia, an ulcer, gallstones, kidney stones, or many other things. Since differentiating between these conditions is often difficult, medical assistance should be obtained.

Summary

When a serious medical problem occurs, it is important to be calm and to provide comfort while taking necessary actions, almost always including obtaining expert medical assistance.

PART FOUR: RESPIRATORY EMERGENCIES

A respiratory emergency occurs when breathing stops as a result of either a disease or an accident. Since the body, particularly the brain, cannot store oxygen, it must have an almost continuous supply. Damage to the brain may occur after a few minutes without oxygen, and death usually occurs in six minutes or less. It is vitally important for artificial respiration to be started as quickly as possible, causing air to flow into and out of a person's lungs.

If a toy, a chunk of food, or other foreign object blocks the airway, it can be a life-or-death emergency. If the foreign object can be easily reached with your fingers, remove it; however, care is necessary to avoid forcing the object deeper into the throat. If the person is coughing, he is still getting some air; if the passage is totally blocked so that he cannot speak or breathe, a true emergency exists.

Stand behind the victim and place your arms around his waist, just above the waist line. Grab your wrist and give the victim a "bear hug" squeeze (fig. 21). The residual air in the lungs will usually pop out the material blocking the air passage. If this does not work, a child may be held upside down and given two or three sharp blows on the upper back. If this is not successful, medical assistance must be obtained quickly.

Other causes of respiratory failure include swelling of the vocal cords (as in croup, asthma, or allergic reactions), swallowing corrosive poisons, breathing air depleted of oxygen (as in the case of carbon monoxide poisoning), electrocution, drowning, heart disease, strangulation, and an overdose of drugs that might depress respiration.

Without oxygen, breath comes shorter and faster; a headache may occur; memory becomes fuzzy, followed by unconsciousness, cyanosis (a bluish tint to lips, tongue, and fingernails), and dilated pupils. Death follows. Even though one is not sure whether the heart is still beating, artificial respiration should be started and should be continued until: (1) the victim begins to breathe for himself; (2) he is pronounced dead by a doctor; (3) he is dead beyond a doubt.

Although there are a number of methods of artificial respiration, research has shown that the mouth-to-mouth method is the most effective. It is the method we will describe. Time is of the essence. It must be started immediately.

- Place the victim on his back.
- Wipe any foreign material from his mouth, using your fingers wrapped in a cloth, if possible, to help trap material and to protect your fingers.
- Tilt the victim's head backward so that his chin is pointing upward (figs. 22 and 23). This helps open the air passage and keeps the tongue from blocking it.

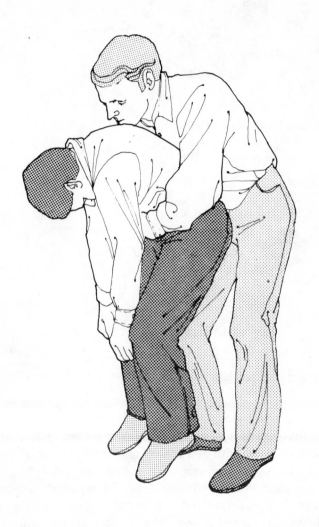

Fig. 21. Giving the victim a "bear hug" squeeze (Heimlicher maneuver)

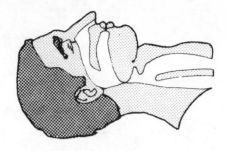

Fig. 22. Placing the victim on his back

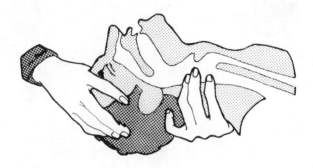

Fig. 23. Opening the air passage

- Unless the victim is a small child or an infant, gently squeeze the victim's nose with the thumb and index finger of hand to prevent leakage of air through the nostrils (fig. 24).
- Give four short breaths initially to see if the patient will breathe on his own; if not, breathe air into his mouth by opening your mouth widely, taking a deep breath, and sealing your mouth tightly around the victim's mouth before you blow. Provide at least one breath every five seconds for an adult—twelve per minute (fig. 25). If the victim is a small child or an infant, cover both mouth and nose with your mouth and give shallow, quick breaths—every three seconds or twenty per minute.

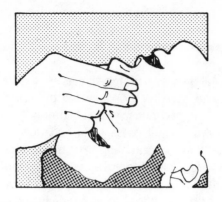

Fig. 24. Pinching the nostrils gently

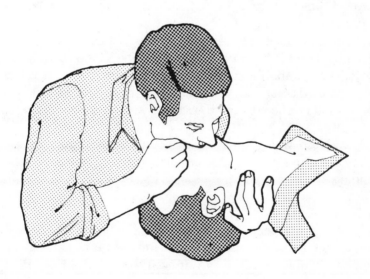

Fig. 25. Sealing your mouth around the victim's mouth

- Watch the victim's chest as you breathe into his mouth. When you see it rise, stop blowing, raise your mouth and turn to the side. (To prevent damaging children's lungs, do not breathe in too much.)
- Listen for exhalation and watch to see the victim's chest fall.
- Repeat the cycle, starting by squeezing the nostrils.
- If there is no air exchange, recheck the victim's head position for obstruction of the air passage. Try again.
- If there is still no air exchange, turn the victim on his side, administer several sharp blows between his shoulder blades over the spine (if he is a child, put him upside down over your arm and give two or three sharp blows between the shoulder blades), clear out foreign matter, and try again.
- If the stomach bulges, turn the victim's head to the side, prepare to clear his mouth, and press your hand briefly and firmly over his rib margin and navel. This may cause regurgitation; if so, clear his mouth. Try breathing again.
- If he starts to breathe, continue to assist him, being careful to match your efforts with his, both in taking in air and in letting it out.

Cardiopulmonary resuscitation is used when the victim is not breathing and his heart has stopped beating. It is a combination of artificial respiration and manual artificial circulation. It is used in cases of cardiac arrest. It does, however, require special training and should not be attempted by those who have never been taught the skill.

Many respiratory emergencies could be prevented by simple safety measures such as not permitting a child to eat while he is running.

PART FIVE: SHOCK

Shock is a reaction of the body to injury. Many vital body functions may be depressed so that life itself is threatened. Sometimes an injured person may not even show signs of shock; or the shock reaction may occur later. Injured victims should be given protective care to prevent the development of shock. Traumatic or injury-related shock is different from electric shock, insulin shock, or anaphalatic shock which will be discussed later.

Most severe injuries will cause shock. Internal or external bleeding; excessive loss of body fluids as in vomiting, diarrhea, or burns;

infections; heart attacks; or poisoning may also cause shock. Chilling, severe pain, and fear may add to the problem.

As shock develops, the skin may become pale or bluish, moist and cool. In dark-complected people it may be necessary to check the nail beds to detect a bluish tinge. Perspiration occurs particularly around the mouth, on the forehead, and in the palms of the hands. The pulse becomes very rapid (over 100) and may be too weak to be felt at the wrist though it can often be felt at the side of the neck. Breathing is usually increased but may be either shallow or deep. Weakness, restlessness and apprehension are common, along with thirst and sometimes nausea and vomiting.

In the later stages of shock the victim may gradually become apathetic and unresponsive. The skin may be mottled and the victim lapse into unconsciousness. The eyes may have a vacant expression and the pupils may be widely dilated. If during unconsciousness the body temperature drops, death may follow.

Emergency protection from shock should be given all victims as soon as the rescuer is assured that breathing is adequate or restored, that bleeding has been stopped, and that the victim has been moved if absolutely necessary:

- The victim should be kept lying down.
- He should be kept covered only enough to prevent the loss of body heat.
- His exact position is determined by the type of injury he has sustained. Where back or neck injuries are suspected, the victim should not be moved unless absolutely necessary.
- Victims who have face and mouth injuries, who are unconscious, or who are vomiting should be placed on their side or at least have their head turned to the side to allow drainage of mouth secretions (fig. 26).

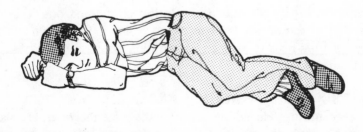

Fig. 26. Placing the victim on his side

- Where breathing is difficult or head injuries are suspected, the victim's head may be raised slightly (fig. 27).

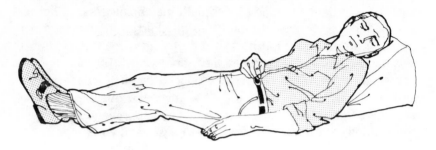

Fig. 27. Raising the victim's head

- If there are no head, back, or neck injuries, the victim's circulation may be improved by raising the victim's feet slightly (fig. 28); when in doubt, keep the victim lying flat.

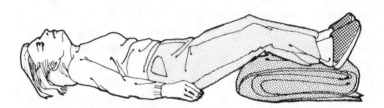

Fig. 28. Raising the victim's feet

- The victim should be given fluids only if no help will be available for an hour or more, if the victim is fully conscious and not vomiting, and if there are no abdominal injuries that might require surgery. A salt-soda solution containing one level teaspoon of salt and ½ level teaspoon of baking soda in a quart of water may help to replace body fluids lost as a result of injury or burns.

PART SIX: CARE OF WOUNDS AND BLEEDING

Every mother deals frequently with wounds. A wound is an injury to the body in which tissue is damaged. Wounds are classified as open wounds, in which skin or mucous membrane is broken, and closed wounds, in which the injury involves the underlying tissues and the skin remains unbroken. These latter are familiar to us as bruises; resulting discoloration is due to broken capillaries beneath the skin. They are very common in all physical activities. A cold compress applied to the area will help to lessen bleeding and swelling, as will elevation of the part injured. If deep injury is suspected, medical attention may be needed.

In this section we will study open wounds and the treatment for bleeding and infections, the two main concerns of the home nurse. The common types of open wounds are described below:

- An abrasion is a scraping or rubbing off of the outer layer of the skin or mucous membrane, such as occurs when a child falls or slides on a rough surface. Since abrasions are superficial and usually do not bleed extensively, infection is a real possibility unless the wound is cleaned adequately with soap and water.

- Punctures are wounds caused by the penetration of a sharp object (such as a nail, an ice pick, a bullet, a spear or an arrow) deep into the underlying body tissues. These wounds usually bleed very little externally but may cause serious internal bleeding and are often subject to infection. They are difficult to cleanse and should be watched closely for signs of infection. A deep puncture wound or one caused by a dirty object should be seen by a doctor. There is danger of tetanus developing in such a wound if the victim is not adequately immunized, and the doctor may wish to give a booster shot for added protection.

- An incision or cut is caused by a sharp object such as a knife, a piece of glass, or a razor blade. (A paper cut is a minor but painful incision.) If the cut is deep, bleeding may be severe, and nerves, muscles, and tendons may be involved. The home nurse should control bleeding and seek medical help; it may be necessary for health personnel to repair the wound with stitches.

- A laceration or tear is a jagged, irregular wound caused by something hard like a rock, a tool, a machine, a bicycle or an automobile. The surrounding tissue is often damaged, and bleeding may be profuse. Infection may be a problem if bacteria are present in the wound. A minor laceraton may be washed with soap and water, but where bleeding is severe, a pressure dressing should be applied and the victim taken to the nearest medical facility.

- An avulsion occurs when tissues are torn from the body (as in the case of bites by an animal or loss of a finger, a leg, or an ear). Any part torn from the victim should be taken to the hospital along with the victim; a surgeon may be able to re-attach the part.

Because a person may bleed to death very rapidly with a major wound, the first-aider must immediately seek to stop such bleeding by using direct pressure over the wound. The best way to do this is to apply a thick pad of cloth over the wound and apply pressure with the palm of the hand on the dressing. In the absence of a thick pad, the hand itself may be used. On the extremities a pressure dressing may be applied. Use a stretchy material such as an elastic bandage or a knit material over the padded wound. The first-aider must be careful not to make the bandage too tight; this would cut off the circulation. After a pressure dressing has been applied, elevate the wounded area above the level of the heart to slow bleeding. If the bandage becomes soaked with blood, add another dressing *without* removing the first one.

A tourniquet is used only when the bleeding cannot be stopped in any other way (such as when an arm or leg has been cut off). Once placed in position, *it should be removed only by a doctor.*

When severe bleeding occurs, the home nurse or first-aider should concentrate on stopping the blood loss, not on cleaning the wound. With minor wounds involving the skin surfaces (such as abrasions, small lacerations, and animal bites), scrubbing with soap and water helps to prevent infection. After the area has been cleansed, blot it dry and apply a sterile dressing. An antiseptic is not necessary if the wound has been adequately cleaned. The home nurse should watch any wound for evidence of infection such as redness, swelling, pus, throbbing pain, red streaks leading from the wound, or fever. If any of these problems occur, quick medical attention should be obtained.

Younger family members should be taught to care for wounds that might occur when no adult is present to help them. Boy scouts in the family can help by teaching other family members what they have learned.

PART SEVEN: POISONING

Almost anything could be a poison under certain circumstances. By definition, any liquid, solid, or gas that interferes with the body's normal functioning is a poison. A substance may be so common and ordinary that precautions are not taken. Aspirin, castor beans, iron tablets, certain plants, and furniture polish are examples of very dangerous common things. Every mother should be aware of safety precautions that can help protect her family from accidental poisoning. Little children are the most likely victims since they may put almost anything they pick up into their mouths. If a mother suspects that someone has eaten a poison, she should find out as much as possible about what has happened, including asking the person and any possible observers. Sometimes children cannot help at all, but sometimes they can provide valuable clues. Locating the container may be very helpful. Also look for burns or stains around the mouth and smell the victim's breath. The symptoms vary with the material ingested. Nothing at all may occur initially; symptoms such as vomiting, choking, pallor, sleepiness, convulsions, unconsciousness, hyperactivity, nausea, or pain may occur—sometimes without an obvious explanation.

When poisoning by mouth is suggested, look into the victim's mouth and remove all tablets, powder, plants or any other material you find. Also examine for cuts, burns, or any unusual coloring. Wipe the mouth out with a cloth; wash it with plain water if necessary. Then call the doctor or poison control center for further advice. The number for the poison control center in your area should be posted near your phone. When you call, identify yourself by name and the poisoning victim by name, age and sex and give your relationship to the victim. Have the package or poison in your hand and identify what the victim took and how much.

If no medical help is immediately available, you will need to decide for yourself what to do.

- Keep calm, there is almost always time enough to think before you act.
- If breathing has stopped, give mouth-to-mouth resuscitation.
- Never cause anyone to vomit if they are unconscious, having convulsions (fits), have swallowed strong corrosives (look for burns around the lips and mouth), or have swallowed petroleum products such as gasoline, kerosene or cleaning fluids.
- If caustic poisons or petroleum products have been swallowed, have the conscious victim drink one to two glassfuls of milk (or water) to dilute the poison.

- Vomiting can be induced by giving syrup of ipecac (3 tsp. followed by a glass of liquid.) This medicine can be purchased from a pharmacist and will keep at room temperature for several years so that it will be available in the event a family member eats a poisonous substance.
- If vomiting is indicated, be certain the victim is in a sitting-up position or a leaning-forward position so that choking on the vomited materials does not occur.
- After the victim has vomited, administer an antidote. If you do not know what the antidote is, use medicinal activated charcoal. This can be purchased from a drugstore and kept with the first-aid supplies. Burned toast is not a substitute for activated charcoal.
- Do not give substances such as alcohol, coffee, or stimulants unless specifically told to do so by the physician.

First Aid for Inhaled Poisons

Inhaled poisons include carbon monoxide, vapors from volatile liquids, compounds from chlorine, and gas from cooling and heating equipment. In every case first aid includes removing the victim from the source and getting him into fresh air while a rescue unit with oxygen is summoned. If breathing has stopped, give mouth-to-mouth resuscitation.

Contact Poisons

Plants such as poison ivy or poison sumac can cause a severe skin reaction. First aid includes removal of contaminated clothing and flushing of the affected area with large quantities of water. Washing with soap and water for at least five minutes will help to remove any irritating substances. In the case of corrosive substances, seek medical help.

Snakebite Poisoning

Snakebites from poisonous snakes are another danger in some areas. The objectives for first aid for snakebites are to reduce the circulation of blood in the bite area, to delay the absorption of venom, to prevent making the local wound worse, and to keep the victim breathing, using mouth-to-mouth resuscitation if necessary. If poisonous snakes are found where you live, be sure family members know the specific first-aid treatment necessary.

- Immobilize the victim's arm or leg in lowered position, keeping the bite area *below* heart level.
- Limit movement.
- Put cold compresses over the wound.
- Get medical help.

For treatment of snakebite away from your area, check with a competent first-aid book.

Miscellaneous Poisoning

In many parts of the world, marine life may be a source of poisoning, either through the eating of poisonous fish or shellfish or through the stings, bites, or bristles of various forms of sea life. Families should contact local government health agencies to determine dangers to be found in their area and should have information in their homes about first-aid measures that may need to be taken.

Insect poisoning is also a problem in most parts of the world. The stings of ants, bees, wasps, hornets, and yellow jackets are annoying and can cause death in people who are allergic to the stings. Multiple stings of certain ants occasionally cause death. The bites or stings of fleas, mosquitoes, lice, gnats, and chiggers are annoying but rarely dangerous except as carriers of disease. Minor bites and stings might be made more comfortable with the application of cold followed by a soothing lotion such as calamine. In the case of a bee sting, remove the stinger.

Severe allergic reactions may cause breathing to stop and the need for artificial mouth-to-mouth resuscitation. A cold application will help to slow circulation in the area of a serious bite. Seek medical help.

Summary

Everyone should be aware of the sources of poisoning in his home and surrounding areas where family members work or play. Remember!
- Suspect poisoning when someone suddenly becomes sick or behaves in an unusual manner and there is no explanation for the illness or abnormal behavior.
- Many things in your home are very poisonous. Check if you're not sure.
- If you take enough of anything, it can be poisonous.

- The most critical period of time is the first hour or two after the poisoning occurs. Do not delay seeking advice.

PART EIGHT: BURNS

Fire and burns continue to be a major safety problem for people of all ages, but especially for children under four and for older people. Heat, radiation, and chemicals are the three general causes of burns. Many burn victims suffer untold agony, disfigurement, and sometimes death. Although burns are classified according to depth or degree of tissue destroyed, it is not always possible to determine the degree of a burn at first. Furthermore, the severity of the burn may vary in different parts of the burned area. When in doubt about the seriousness of a burn, obtain medical help.

First-degree burns are characterized by reddening of the skin accompanied by mild swelling and pain. They may result from sun or brief contact with hot objects, hot water, or steam. These burns usually heal rapidly since damage is limited to the outer layer of the skin. To relieve the pain, place the burned area in cold water or hold it under running water. This eliminates the heat. A dry dressing may be applied after the area has been cooled.

Second-degree burns are accompanied by blisters along with redness. The heat has penetrated more deeply and causes body fluids to collect beneath the skin. This type of burn may be caused by contact with hot liquids or steam, flash burns from gasoline or kerosene, and sometimes by a severe sunburn. Second-degree burns are quite painful.

The treatment of small second-degree burns is similar to the treatment of first-degree burns. Immersing the burned part in cold water reduces the burning effect and helps prevent additional damage to deeper layers. Avoid breaking the blisters as this may introduce infection. With a severe burn which requires medical attention, it is best not to apply any ointment, spray, or home remedy. A dry sterile gauze dressing may be helpful as a protective covering while enroute to medical care. If legs or feet are badly burned, they should be kept elevated and at rest.

Third-degree burns penetrate through all layers of the skin causing deeper destruction. Third-degree burns may be caused by flame-ignited clothing, immersion in very hot water, or by contact with hot objects or electricity. Most serious burns involve all three types of burn, and it may be difficult for the first-aider to determine which is which. Serious burns of the hands, feet, or face or burns covering large areas of the body should receive prompt medical attention. When a large area of skin surface is destroyed, much body fluid is lost, and the possibility of infection is great. Shock is almost always present with extensive burns.

Treatment for third-degree burns includes treatment for shock, protection from infection, and getting the victim to medical help as quickly as possible. Do not try to remove charred clothing which is stuck. If it will not delay reaching medical care, cover the whole burned area with a sterile dressing or freshly laundered sheet. If feet or legs are involved, keep them elevated and do not allow the victim to walk about. If the hands are involved, keep them elevated higher than the heart. Persons with facial burns should sit up and should be watched for difficulty in breathing. If the victim is conscious and not nauseated, encourage him to sip some broth, a soft drink, or a weak salt and soda solution (1 teaspoon salt and ½ teaspoon baking soda in a quart of water neither hot nor cold). Give frequent reassurance to help counteract anxiety about what is happening. A cold pack may be applied to a burned face, hands, or feet. Do not put any ointment, commercial burn preparation, or home remedy on serious burns.

If strong acids or alkalies come in contact with any part of the body, chemical burns may result. First aid consists of removing the substance as quickly as possible with large quantities of water. This is more important than trying to neutralize the chemical. Continue rinsing the area for at least five minutes. Acid or alkaline burns of the eye should be treated by rinsing with large quantities of plain water. Have the victim lie on his side, hold the eyelid open and pour water from the inner corner of the eye outward. Be sure the victim is seen by medical personnel, since burns, particularly alkaline ones, tend to be progressively injurious, and eyesight may be lost.

Although sunburn rarely requires hospitalization, it is often accompanied by great discomfort which may include fever and headache. The development of such symptoms usually takes from four to fifteen hours. First-aid measures are the same as for other first- and second-degree burns. Medical help should be sought for sunburn covering ten to fifteen percent of the body. In such cases, do not put any ointment on the sunburn before seeing the doctor.

Summary

Family members should be taught the basic first-aid principles for burns, but even more important is a family discussion of ways to prevent burns from happening. Consider showing pictures of degrees of burns and washing chemicals out of the eyes.

PART NINE: BONE AND JOINT INJURIES

Every mother soon learns that injuries to the bones, ligaments, tendons, and muscles are very common. Occasionally such an injury is serious enough to cause lasting disability, especially if it is not properly treated. These injuries occur at work, at play, in the home, and especially in or by moving vehicles.

When excessive force overstretches or overexerts a muscle, a strain may occur. If the force continues and stretches the joint attachments (ligaments and tendons), a sprain may result. The hurting is usually sudden and severe at first but subsides more rapidly than in fractures or dislocations.

Cold is applied first to the injured part; it alleviates pain and prevents swelling. Rest and elevation are used for the various types of injuries. Attempt to keep the injured part comfortably elevated above the level of the heart. Gentle splinting with a pillow or elastic bandage is often helpful. Whereas cold is used as an initial first aid treatment, heat may be more comfortable after the first day or so.

A dislocation occurs when the end of a bone is displaced at the joint. With the dislocation there is usually marked deformity, swelling, and pain. Sometimes a snap or pop is heard or felt at the moment of injury. Fingers are frequently dislocated as well as are the shoulder, jaw, toes, elbow, and knee joints. Muscles, blood vessels, and nerves in the area may be injured. First aid includes immobilizing the area and seeking medical help. Usually a joint remains swollen and painful for some time, even after the dislocation has been corrected.

A fracture is a break or crack in the bone. A closed (or simple) fracture means the skin has not been broken. If the skin has been broken along with the bone, the fracture is said to be open or compound. The most common causes of fractures are motor vehicle accidents, falls, and accidents related to recreational and sports activities. It is often difficult to know without an X-ray if a fracture exists. But some simple clues that suggest a fracture in-

134

clude pain and tenderness, hearing a bone snap, or feeling a grating sensation. Other signs include swelling, obvious deformities, and pain when the area of the injury is touched.

"Splint them where they lie" is the rule. If the injured person is conscious, he may be able to help the first-aider position the injured part in the most comfortable position. If unconscious, the person with an obvious fracture must be handled as any other unconscious victim—with extreme caution. Make certain breathing is adequate and treat for shock. Protect the head and neck from further injury. Stop obvious bleeding by direct pressure on the wound with a sterile (if available) dressing. If nothing sterile is available, use the cleanest cloth within reach. The person's own clothing will do. Obtain help immediately from the best medical source.

If bone ends protrude through broken skin, treat as any other wound to prevent infection. The first-aider should not attempt to set (reduce) fractures or dislocations.

Splinting limbs and rigging rigid supports for the spine and trunk in victims is necessary before attempting movement. Splint devices are used to immobilize a part when a fracture or dislocation is suspected; they protect the part from further injury and help reduce the pain. A simple form of splinting is to pad the area and then tie or tape it to another area. This can be done by taping legs together or by binding an injured arm to the chest or side. Boards, canes, sticks, rolled up blankets or newspapers, and cardboard are other items that can be used as splints. They should be padded to protect the body part and should be long enough to extend past the joints on either side of the suspected fracture. Belts, ties, handkerchiefs, or strips of torn cloth can be used to tie the splints in place. Be sure the splints are not too tight, and where possible, use cold and elevation for prevention of swelling, as in minor injuries.

A blow on the head may or may not cause a skull fracture. Actually, even without a skull fracture there may be a serious injury in the brain. The biggest problem is bleeding inside the skull itself. Loss of consciousness may be either immediate or delayed.

A person who has received a severe blow to the head should receive medical attention and should be watched closely for twenty-four to forty-eight hours, since bleeding in the area of the brain might cause symptoms to develop belatedly. Vomiting, paralysis, disturbances of speech, bleeding from the nose, ear canal, or mouth, convulsions, headache and/or dizziness, unconsciousness, or unequal size of the pupils of the eyes are all indications that further medical attention is needed. Minor scalp wounds bleed profusely but in themselves do not indicate damage to the brain. The bleeding can usually be controlled by applying direct pressure while medical attention is obtained to suture the laceration.

Summary

Bone and joint injuries may involve a great deal of pain and discomfort. Comforting reassurance helps allay fear and shock. Splinting may provide some relief of pain along with reducing further injury. Knowing what to do and what not to do is of great importance.

PART TEN: EYES, EARS, NOSE, AND MOUTH

Nosebleeds, earaches, and foreign objects in the eye are common emergencies. In this chapter we will consider problems in each of these areas.

Eyes

■ Specks of dust and dirt which often get in the eye are painful but not usually serious. On the other hand, metallic particles can be very damaging. Pulling the upper eyelid down over the lower lid will cause the tears to flow, and soft particles will often be washed out. If the foreign object can be seen, it may be removed with the corner of a clean handkerchief. Never use anything blunt such as a match or toothpick. If the particle cannot be located and does not wash away with the tears, depress the upper lid with a matchstick or similar object (fig. 29) and evert the eyelid by pulling the lashes upward (fig. 30). There the particle can be washed out with water or removed with the corner of a clean handkerchief. If pain and discomfort continue, the eye may have been scratched, or a foreign object may be embedded in it. Place a dry compress over the closed eye and seek medical help. The dressing will help to prevent the victim from rubbing his eye, increasing the damage.

■ The eyes are subject to many types of injury, including sunburn and blunt or penetrating injuries. A black eye may indicate damage to the soft tissues of the eye as a result of a severe blow.

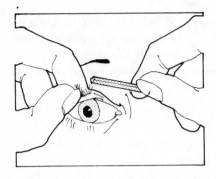 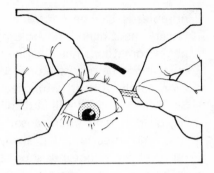

Fig. 29. Depressing the upper lid   **Fig. 30. Everting the eyelid**

Since blindness may result from serious eye injuries, medical help should be sought as soon as possible whenever there is a question about the seriousness of the problem.

Ears

- A foreign object in an ear can be extremely uncomfortable. Prodding with a matchstick, hairpin, or sharp object may create a bigger problem. Medical attention usually is necessary to remove foreign objects from the ear. When an insect flies into the ear, the noise may be very annoying. Putting a few drops of warm mineral or olive oil in the affected ear usually kills the insect. Sometimes when the person tilts his head to the side the oil and insect drain out.

- Earaches can be extremely painful and usually occur because of increased pressure or because of a middle-ear infection. Yawning, chewing gum, or swallowing may relieve pressure changes, but middle-ear infection should be treated by medical personnel to prevent serious complications.

- Perforation (breaking) of the eardrum may occur as a result of an infection, a blow to the head, sudden extreme noises such as blasting, or deep diving. Drainage from the ear might indicate rupture of the eardrum; medical help should be obtained.

Nose

- Nosebleeds can result from injury, infection, allergy, a change in altitude, or from other problems. Most are minimal in amount and duration, but others are extensive. The great majority of nosebleeds can be controlled by grasping the nose firmly between the fingers and holding it for five to ten minutes. Ice packs sometimes help, applied along with the pressure. If bleeding cannot be controlled, obviously medical attention is necessary. Apply pressure while getting the victim to the doctor.

- Sometimes a child will stuff paper or a bean into his nose. If not removed it may swell, absorb moisture, and may cause a foul odor and infection. It is always best to have the foreign matter removed by a doctor as soon as possible after it is discovered.
- A broken nose sometimes occurs as a result of a blow. It is usually obvious because of the distortion of the nose and the difficulty the victim experiences in breathing due to the swelling. No first-aid measures are needed, but like all fractures, medical help should be sought.

Mouth

- Mouth injuries are frequent and usually heal readily if they are minor. When a tooth has been pulled, the bleeding can usually be controlled by pressure in the area with a small piece of gauze. Large lacerations in the mouth or on the tongue sometimes need to be sutured.
- Fractures of the face and jaw are common in motor vehicle accidents or in other types of violent injuries. There is often extreme pain and severe hemorrhage. The victim will have difficulty opening his mouth or speaking. First aid includes: clearing any debris such as broken teeth from the mouth, making sure the victim is breathing regularly, having the victim's head and shoulders elevated, and making sure that secretions drain from the mouth. Medical help will be necessary.

Summary

Sight, hearing, smell, and taste are vitally important functions of our bodies, and the organs involved should be protected so that we can live and enjoy life completely.

PART ELEVEN: RESCUE AND TRANSPORTATION

In most disabling accidents the victim must be moved. The way in which it is done may endanger the victim's life if proper care is not taken. An injured person should not be hastily picked up and taken to the doctor until the extent of his injuries has been determined. Although in some situations speed is essential, in most cases the victim can be treated where he is until help arrives or until airway obstruction and hemorrhage are cared for, fractures are splinted, and the victim has been reassured.

Immediate action is necessary in the following situations:
- Fire, danger of fire, or explosion
- Danger of asphyxia due to lack of oxygen or to gas
- Serious traffic hazards
- Drowning
- Exposure to cold, intense heat, or intense weather conditions
- Possibility of injury due to collapsing walls or buildings
- Electrical injury or potential injury
- Pinning by heavy equipment or materials

It is difficult to lift or carry an injured person gently and safely. If a person must be dragged to safety, he should be pulled by the shoulders, and his body should not be twisted. A blanket, board, or rug under the patient may simplify pulling. This is a good method to use if the victim has no injuries but is being rescued from fire, smoke, or gas inhalation and if he is too big for the first-aider to lift (fig. 31).

A good method for a victim of minor injuries who can partially help himself is the one shown in figure 32. Have the victim place his good arm across your shoulder. Hold his wrist with your hand. If necessary, encircle the victim's waist with your free hand to offer support on the other side. Walk slowly and carefully, preferably in step with the victim.

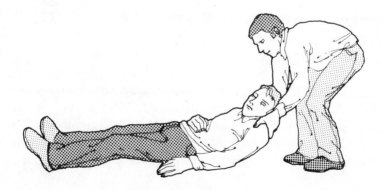

Fig. 31. Pulling the victim by the shoulders

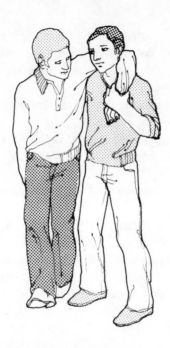

Fig. 32. Letting the victim help himself walk

A child or lightweight adult can be picked up and carried as shown in figure 33. If two people are available, a chair may be used to carry a victim who has no neck, back, or leg injuries. It is a good method for going through narrow halls or up and down stairs.

Two people can form a seat with their hands grasping each others' wrists to carry a patient who can help by placing his arms around their shoulders (fig. 34).

Where several people are available, a blanket or sheet or just the helpers' hands may be used to carry a victim. The helpers work from both sides, with one person holding the victim's head steady. One person must be in charge of calling "signals" so that all the helpers lift together and move together; otherwise, the victim may be injured by unnecessary and uncoordinated movement. Litters can be improvised with two poles or sticks and a blanket or jackets.

If neck or back injuries have occurred, the victim should not be moved unless his life is in danger where he is.

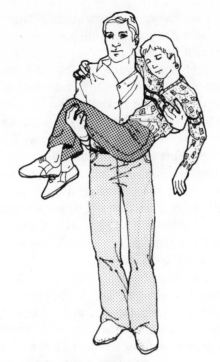

Fig. 33. Carrying a child or lightweight adult

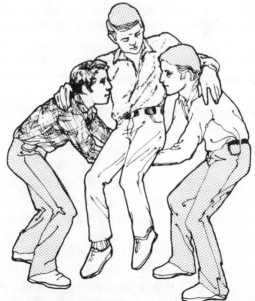

Fig. 34. Forming a seat for the victim

When a victim is in danger of electrocution from contact with electrical current, he must not be touched by the rescuer, since this allows the current to pass through the body of the rescuer also. First, disconnect the current or shut off the main power source if this is possible. If the current cannot be shut off, a loop of dry rope or cloth around the victim's hand or boot may be used to drag him away from the current. A dry, non-conducting pole or board may also be used to push the victim away from the power source. If the rescuer must use his hand, it should be protected by rubber, layers of heavy paper, or cloth. A roll of newspapers may be used to push the source of current away from the victim.

Do not attempt to rescue a victim from an oxygen-deficient atmosphere until ventilation is restored. Exhaust fumes and poisonous gas work very quickly, and you can be affected while attempting rescue in a closed area.

To rescue someone in a burning building, place a thick, wet cloth over your mouth and nose. This will protect you from heat but not from poisonous gases. Do not open a door that is hot to the touch. Use stairways rather than elevators. If there is smoke, crawl along the floor where more oxygen is available.

Water rescue can often be effected by throwing a rope, a pole, or a cloth to the victim while you hold the other end. Do not attempt a swimming rescue unless you have been trained in life-saving. Many drowning victims must be given mouth-to-mouth resuscitation to restore breathing.

Remember that in rescuing a person from a car it may be necessary to break the windows or remove the doors. Be careful that the victim is not injured further by flying glass.

Summary

In rescue situations, thinking through the situation quickly is the first step. As with other first-aid measures, it is important to avoid adding to the problem. Knowing what to do and how to do it may prevent untold suffering. Family members need to know what to do in their home when an emergency rescue is necessary.

PART TWELVE: ENVIRONMENTAL EXCESSES

Both heat and cold in excess can do damage to the human body, whose temperature is expected to remain relatively constant regardless of the surroundings. The effect of either heat or cold is influenced by such factors as the length of exposure, temperature, humidity, and wind.

Heatstroke

Let us first consider heatstroke (sunstroke). This can be caused by either excessive heat or too much exposure to the direct rays of the sun. Sometimes the body mechanism for regulating temperature seems to go astray and the body temperature rises swiftly and dangerously, even up to 106° F or higher. The skin is hot, dry, and red with no evidence of perspiration. Medical help should be sought at once. In the meantime, measures should be taken to reduce the body temperature immediately. This can be done by sponging the skin surfaces with a mixture of water and alcohol, applying cold packs continuously, especially to the head, or by placing the victim in a tub of cool water (with no ice in the water) until the victim's temperature is lowered to 102° F. This usually takes fifteen to twenty minutes. Remove him from the tub, dry him, and allow him to rest in a cool place. Check his temperature at intervals to be sure it does not begin to rise again.

Heat Cramps

Heat cramps are caused by a deficiency of both salt and water due to profuse sweating. The cramps usually affect the muscles of the legs and the abdomen. This problem is often found in athletes working out in hot weather. Because they are perspiring freely, their bodies are losing both salt and water in large amounts. The cramps occur when the salt is not replaced. In addition to the cramps, the victim may feel weak, nauseated, dizzy, and faint. He is pale and perspiring, but his body temperature is normal. First-aid treatment consists of firm pressure and massage on the cramped muscles and sips of salt water, one teaspoon of salt per glass, to be consumed over a period of thirty minutes.

Heat Exhaustion

Heat exhaustion (also called heat prostration) is found most commonly in places where individuals are working for long periods where the temperature and humidity are both high. Kitchens, laundries, and canneries lacking airconditioning often foster heat exhaustion. As with heat cramps, the problem occurs because the body loses large amounts of salt and water. The victim has approximately a normal body temperature, but complains of being weak, dizzy, faint, and nauseated. He may vomit. His skin is pale and clammy. The treatment is similar to that for heat cramps—salt water. In addition, have the victim lie down with his feet slightly elevated. Apply cool, wet cloths to his face. He should rest for several hours and should be protected from exposure to abnormally warm temperatures. Medical care may be necessary if the victim is vomiting or does not recover promptly.

Frostbite

Frostbite is, of course, a problem in only some parts of the world. It occurs when parts of the body are exposed to temperatures low enough to cause ice crystals to form in and around the cells. The nose, ears, fingers, and toes are most susceptible to frostbite. Freezing is accelerated by wind and long exposure. Persons who smoke have much more difficulty with frostbite because they have less efficient circulation. Before frostbite occurs, the area may appear flushed; then a tingling sensation occurs, followed by pain. As the ice crystals form, the skin appears greyish-yellow and glossy. The victim feels numbness in the area; eventually blisters may appear. It is best to rewarm the frozen part quickly by submerging it in warm (102° to 103° F) water. The warm temperature can be tested by submerging your forearm in the water. The water should feel warm but not hot to your forearm. *Never rub the frozen area, since this creates cell damage.* Discontinue the warming when the area becomes flushed. Severe swelling may develop. Never break the blisters. Cover the area as for burns if the victim is to be transported. Do not allow the victim to walk if the feet or legs are affected. Give the victim fluids as in the case of burns—sips of one teaspoon table salt and ½ teaspoon baking soda per one quart of water. Frostbite may often be prevented by a person's wearing loose, warm clothing. Frequent changes of gloves and socks are wise when working or playing in the cold to keep them dry.

Snowburn

Snowburn is caused by the reflection of the sun on snow. The eyes may be temporarily blinded by snowburn. Pain may develop several hours after exposure. Both the eyes and skin should be protected from snowburn. If a burn does occur, it should be

144

treated in the same way as sunburn.

Mothers should help family members learn to protect themselves from excesses of either heat or cold. They should know how to care for emergencies that arise as a result of excessive heat or cold when they are away from home.

IMPROVISED EQUIPMENT

Throughout the previous chapters, mention has been made about using improvised equipment. The newspaper bag and the accessory bag have already been described. In this chapter we will suggest a number of ways to improvise other needed equipment. Every home nurse will also find ways of creating her own useful nursing aids. They will vary from home to home and from patient to patient. Rarely can improvised equipment compete with its commercial counterpart, but for short-term illness it has the advantage of economy and availability. When families are dealing with long-term illness, they may wish to rent or buy professional hospital equipment.

ELEVATING THE BED
    The ways to elevate the bed to the hip level (approximately 30 to 32 inches from the floor) of the home nurse include:
- Adding an extra mattress.
- Filling # 10 cans or buckets with sand or soil, making sure all of the cans are at the same level, then placing the lids or a piece of wood on top of the substance in the can to prevent the bed-legs from sinking into the sand; removing the casters to prevent the bed from sliding.
- Using stacks of books, magazines or newspapers tied securely together and placed under each bed leg, cutting a round hole in the top few layers of newspapers to hold the bed leg, then removing the casters.
- Using kitchen chairs, two at the head of the bed and two at the foot (if the rails at the head and foot of the bed are even).
- Using cinder blocks but being careful not to bump the shins.
- Using wooden blocks cut 8x8x12 inches (figs. 35 and 36).

SPECIAL EQUIPMENT FOR THE BED
- A foot support should be approximately 2 inches higher than the patient's toes and should be braced against the foot of the bed. It can be made from a strong card box 9x12x14 inches.

147

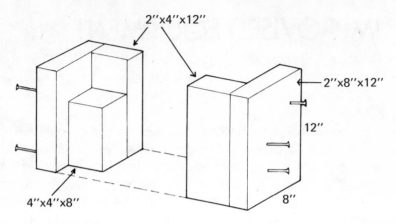

Fig. 35. Assembling the wooden block

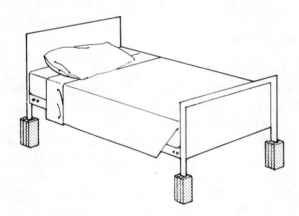

Fig. 36. Elevating the bed with wooden blocks

Tape the cover shut so the box is more sturdy, and cover it with contact paper to make the surface washable. The footboard not only allows the patient's feet to be in a normal position, but also keeps the weight of the covers off the patient's toes.

- A box 10x12x24 inches cut like the bed table and placed over the feet can also serve to keep the covers from touching the patient's toes.
- It is difficult to elongate the bed for the tall patient, though if the bed is open-ended, two chairs may be placed at the end, and foam padding or folded blankets may be used to bring the level of the chairs' seats to that of the bed. A piece of padded board

slipped under the foot of the mattress may also work to extend the mattress. The problem of making the bedding long enough is less easily solved.

■ With a confused patient, bed rails may be desirable. The commercial rails used on hospital beds can be raised and lowered and are easily used. Improvised ones include boards tied to the head and foot of the bed (fig. 37) or kitchen chairs tied together alongside the bed (fig. 38).

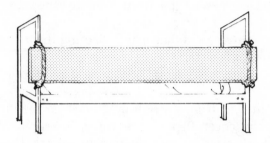

Fig. 37. Board rail, tied to head and foot boards of bed

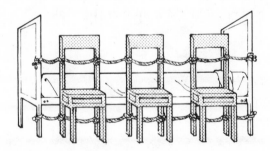

Fig. 38. Kitchen chairs tied together as a rail

■ A rope tied to the foot of the bed gives the patient a means of pulling himself to a sitting position.

BACKRESTS
Various backrests include:
■ A card table tilted against the head of the bed. A table leaf or wide piece of wood could also be used in this manner.

149

- Commercial backrests with armrests.
- A cushion from a chair or lounge or a wedge-shaped pillow.
- An inverted chair against which pillows are placed. Removing the legs from the chair may help.
- A cardboard box. This makes one of the nicest backrests. Choose a box about 24x24x18 inches that has the cover flaps still on it. The procedure is as follows:
  - The broad side of the carton will be the sloping part of the backrest. It should be at least 24 inches wide.
  - Slit the corners of the front side from top to bottom (fig. 39).
  - Fold the two sides diagonally. Scoring them first will facilitate the folding (fig. 40).
  - Bend inward any excess cardboard at the top and sides (fig. 41).
  - Bring the cut front portion up to rest on the diagonal sides. Bring the cover flap of the carton down to complete the sloped side against which the patient will rest (fig. 42).
  - If desired, the box can be covered with material or contact paper (the latter makes it washable). Use of a piece of foam under a covering made of quilted fabric allows the backrest to be used without extra pillows (fig. 43).

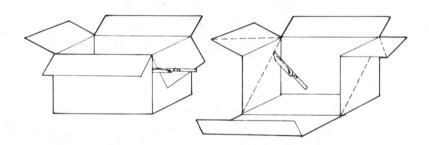

Fig. 39. Slitting corners of the box   **Fig. 40. Scoring the sides of the box**

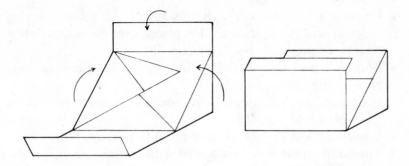

Fig. 41. Bending inward excess cardboard

Fig. 42. Bringing front portion up and cover flap down

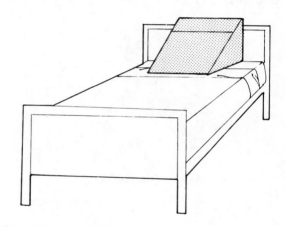

Fig. 43. Carton as a backrest

OVERBED TABLES

Overbed tables can be improvised in the following ways:

- Place the free end of an ironing board across the bed. One which is adjustable in height works best.
- Use a wooden crate or box from which the long sides have been removed.
- Place a board on several large books or on two block of wood.
- Partially cut off the legs of a card table.
- Make an overbed table from a heavy cardboard box 10x12x24 inches (fig. 44).

- Remove the top flaps.
- Partially cut out the two long sides of the carton, leaving room enough so that when it is placed over the patient's legs he is not completely restricted (fig. 45).
- Choose a box that will allow him to rest his arms comfortably on the top of the table.
- If desired, cut hand holds in the ends to allow you to pick up the table easily (fig. 46).
- Covering the cut edges will give stability to the table.
- The whole table may be covered with contact paper, but the eating surface at least should be covered to allow the area to be washable. Some mothers cover the top with blank newsprint to give their child a writing and drawing surface. A new piece is put on when necessary.

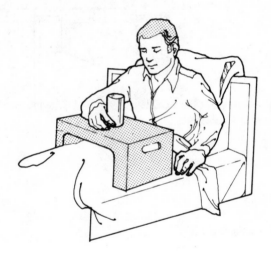

Fig. 44. Overbed table made from a heavy cardboard box

EQUIPMENT FOR BODY DISCHARGES

- A bedpad under the patient may be desirable when he uses the bedpan. One can be made from newspapers about 15x23 inches covered by old sheeting about 25x36 inches. The paper is laid in the center of the cloth, and the overlap material forms corners that can be basted or pinned. A sheet of plastic along with the newspapers will make the bedpad waterproof.
- Almost any container that will hold water may be used as a

urinal. A tall fruit can would work well, but be sure there are no sharp or rough edges when the lid is removed.

- A bedpan is almost impossible to improvise satisfactorily. In an emergency a flat pan about 2x8x12 inches can be placed in a cardboard box and a hole cut in the middle. It is almost impossible, however, to find a cardboard box heavy enough to bear the weight of the buttocks, and if the pan is aluminum, it also may be bent out of shape.

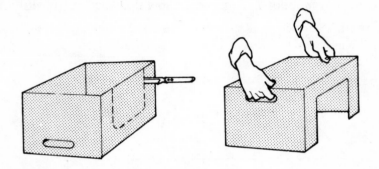

Fig. 45. Partially cutting out the two long sides of a carton

Fig. 46. Cutting hand holds

- A commode can be made from an old chair (fig. 47).

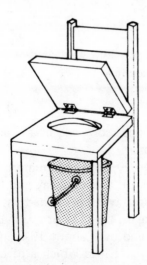

Fig. 47. A commode made from an old chair

MISCELLANEOUS EQUIPMENT

- Door silencers can be made in the following ways:
  - Tear a 3x24-inch piece of fabric lengthwise toward the center to form 1½x10-inch ties and a 2-inch center section. The center is placed across the door latch, and the tails are tied around the knob on each side.
  - A piece of innertube 3x10 inches can be used. Cut a slit near each end to slip over the door knob on each side of the door.
- When traveling, you may need a paper cup. Take a square of clean paper about 7x7 inches. Follow the diagram (fig. 48).

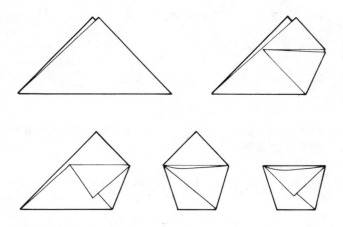

Fig. 48. How to fold a paper cup

- We mentioned the accessory bag in an earlier chapter, but here are the full directions.
  - Use a piece of heavy, washable material about 28x20 inches.
  - Lay the material out the long way and fold up one end about 6 inches. This area will be divided into pockets of varying widths depending on the patient's wishes (fig. 49).
  - Fold the other end over about 10 inches and sew the sides. This creates a pocket into which a piece of heavy cardboard can be inserted to make the bag more stable.

154

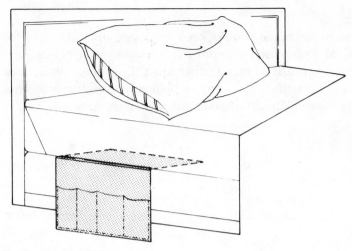

Fig. 49. Pockets in bed bag

- To relieve pressure areas on the elbows or heels, donuts can be made of cotton batting or foam rubber. These should be wrapped with gauze bandages to help them retain their shape and to allow some absorbency. A larger donut for under the buttocks could be improvised from a pillow in which the padding is forced to the sides, and a circle is stitched in the center where a hole can be cut.
- A book rack can be made from a wire coat hanger, as pictured (fig. 50). This, however, would work the most satisfactorily when suspended from a regular, slanted, hospital overbed table.

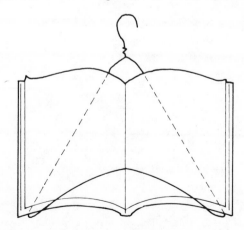

Fig. 50. Book rack made from a wire coat hanger

Summary

The home nurse should keep her eyes and ears open for new kinds of improvised equipment. Thought, imagination, and creativity can result in many other ideas. Challenge family members to come up with suggestions to help solve specific problems. The family handyman can often create special equipment.

BIBLIOGRAPHY

The American National Red Cross. *Advanced First Aid & Emergency Care*. New York: Doubleday & Co., 1973.

Christopherson, Victor. *Rehabilitation Nursing*. New York: McGraw-Hill, 1974.

The Equitable Life Assurance Company. *Home Health Emergencies*. New York: The Equitable Life Assurance Society, 1960.

Fonlara, Vincent J., M.D. *A Parent's Guide to Child Safety*. New York: Thomas Y. Crowell Co., 1973.

Hall, Joanne E., ed. *Nursing the Family in Crisis*. Philadelphia: J. B. Lippincott Co., 1974.

Paxman, Monroe J. and Shirley. *To Bed, to Bed, the Doctor Said*. Walnut Grove, California: Evergreen Press, 1975.

Red Cross Home Nursing Textbook. New York: Doubleday & Co., 1963.

Relief Society Courses of Study (Family Health Lessons). Salt Lake City: The Church of Jesus Christ of Latter-day Saints, 1974, 1975, 1976.

Ross, Elisabeth Kubler. *On Death and Dying*. New York: Macmillan Co., 1969.

Ruslink, Doris. *Family Health and Home Nursing*. New York: Macmillan Co., 1963.

Smith, Dorothy. *Care of the Adult Patient*. Philadelphia: J. B. Lippincott Co., 1963.

Stolten, Jan Henry. *The Health Aid*. Boston: Little, Brown and Co., 1972.

U.S., Department of Agriculture, "Family Food Stockpile for Survival," Home and Garden Bulletin, no. 77.

U.S. Department of Defense, Office of Civil Defense. *In Time of Emergency*, March 1968.

GLOSSARY

Abrasion—a rubbing or scraping away of the skin.

Abscess—a localized collection of pus in the body.

Acute—having severe symptoms of short duration.

Allergic reaction—an abnormal reaction to a substance such as pollens, foods, or medications.

Ambulatory—not bedridden, able to be up and about.

Anemia—a reduction in the number of red blood cells or the hemoglobin content in the blood or both.

Antibody—a substance in the blood that reacts against a foreign substance introduced into the body.

Antidote—any agent administered to prevent or counteract a poison.

Anus—the outlet of the rectum.

Apnea—a time when breathing is suspended.

Artery—a vessel carrying blood away from the heart.

Atrophy—wasting away of a part.

Axilla—armpit.

Bacteria—microscopic organisms larger than viruses.

Bladder—organ which collects urine.

Bland diet—soft, without spice or roughage.

Blood pressure—the pressure within the arteries.

Bruise—an injury causing discoloration under the unbroken skin.

Buttocks—fleshy parts of the back covering the hip joints.

Cardiac—pertaining to the heart.

Carrier—a person who seems well but who can spread disease because he harbors the microorganism.

Cathartic—a medicine used to produce evacuation of the bowels. Also called laxative or purgative.

Catheterize—to introduce a sterile tube into the bladder to withdraw urine.

Chill—a sensation of cold accompanied by shivering. Often occurs initially with the beginning of a serious infection prior to a sharp rise in body temperature.

Chronic—of lengthy duration.

Circulatory system—movement of the blood through the heart, veins, arteries, and capillaries.

Clavicle—the collarbone.

Clinical thermometer—a type of thermometer used to measure body temperature.

Coma—a state of unconsciousness.

Commode—a toilet chair with a removable waste basin. To be used at the bedside.

Communicable disease—transmissible from one person to another.

Compound fracture—a broken bone protruding through the skin.

Concussion—produced by a fall or blow to the head. May produce unconsciousness, pallor, headache, vomiting, or other symptoms.

Constipation—a condition in which the bowels are evacuated with difficulty.

Contamination— the presence of germs.

Contracture—a shortened deformed muscle.

Contusion—another term for bruise.

Convulsion—involuntary spasms or contractions of the large muscles.

Cyanosis—blueness of the skin due to lack of oxygen.

Cystitis—inflammation of the bladder.

Cystoscope—instrument used to examine the interior of the urinary system.

Debilitated—weakened condition.

Decubitus ulcer—pressure sore or bedsore.

Defecation—the discharge of fecal material.

Dehydration—a condition resulting from severe loss of fluid from the body.

Depression—a state of morbid unhappiness.

Dermatitis—an inflammation of the skin.

Diabetes—a disease caused by the inability of the body to produce enough insulin.

Diagnosis—a decision as to the nature of the disease.

Diarrhea—frequent, more or less fluid stools.

Dislocation—the displacement of a bone.

Disoriented—mentally confused.

Dysentery—severe diarrhea.

Dyspnea—difficult or labored breathing.

Dysuria—difficult or painful urination.

Edema—an accumulation of fluid in the tissues.

Emaciated—very thin, wasted.

Emesis—the act of vomiting.

Emetic—a medicine causing vomiting.

Enema—a rectal injection usually used to cleanse the lower bowel.

Epilepsy—a nervous disease marked by convulsions.

Epidemic—unusual prevalence of a disease over a wide area.

Eruption—lesions on the skin, a rash.

Excrete—to discharge waste materials.

Exudate—the serous material that collects in the tissues when inflammation or injury is present.

Feces—the excretion from the bowels.

Flatus—intestinal gas.

Fracture—the breaking of a bone.

Gamma globulin—the part of the human blood plasma containing disease-fighting antibodies.

Gangrene—decay of tissue in a part of the body due to lack of blood supply because of disease or injury.

Gastric—pertaining to the stomach.

Genitalia—the external organs of reproduction in either the male or female.

Groin—the depression between the abdomen and thigh. Also called the inguinal region.

Gynecology—the study of female reproduction, sex organs, and their diseases.

Hallucination—a false sense perception.

Hematoma—a darkened area of the skin, underneath which there is blood.

Hemiplegia—a paralysis of one side of the body.

Hemoglobin—the red matter of the red blood cells which carries oxygen to the tissues and carbon dioxide to the lungs.

Hemorrhage—the escape of blood from a blood vessel.

Hemorrhoid ("piles")—Varicose veins of the anus or rectum.

Hernia—a weakness in a muscle wall that allows an inner body part to slip through.

Hormone—any of a number of chemical compounds in the body having a regulatory effect on other cells remote from them.

Host—the organic body upon or in which parasites live.

Hydrotherapy—treatment by water.

Hypodermic—injection under the skin.

Incision—a wound caused by a cutting instrument.

Immunization—the process of making one less susceptible to a disease.

Impaction—a hard, firm mass of stool lodged near the rectum which cannot be expelled normally by the patient.

Incontinence—inability to control elimination of urine or feces.

Infection—the invasion of body tissues by disease organisms.

Inflammation—the reaction of tissues to injury or infection resulting in heat, swelling, redness, and pain.

Ingestion—taking substances into the body.

Inhalation—breathing in of air.

Inspiration—the drawing in of a breath.

Isolation—the separation of a person from others.

Jaundice—yellowness of the skin and eyes.

Laryngitis—inflammation of the larynx.

Larynx—the voice box.

Laxative—a mild cathartic, an agent to loosen the bowels.

Malaise—a general feeling of illness, tiredness, restlessness, and discomfort.

Metabolism—the chemical changes in the body that produce energy.

Microorganism—microscopic plant or animal.

Mucus—a viscid liquid secreated by the mucous glands located in various parts of the body.

Narcotic—a drug that produces stupor or deep sleep.

Nausea—a feeling of discomfort in the area of the stomach with a tendency to vomit.

Nebulizer—same as an atomizer.

Obsession—an imperative idea difficult to remove in spite of conscious attempts to do so.

Obstetrics—branch of medicine that cares for women during pregnancy, labor, and puerperium (period following childbirth).

Pain threshold—the lower limit of pain capable of producing a response.

Pallor—paleness.

Passive exercise—the movement of a person's body by another person or machine.

Patent medicine—a trade-marked medical preparation sold over the counter without a doctor's order.

Pediatrician—a specialist in children's diseases.

Peristalsis—the wavelike motion of the walls of the digestive tract that carries food along the alimentary canal.

Physiotheraphy—treatment with heat, massage, and manipulation.

Pica—a desire or craving for strange foods or substances like dirt, hair, leaves, or sand.

Plasma—the fluid portion of the blood in which the red cells, white cells, and platelets are suspended.

Posterior—back.

Pressure sores—bed sores or decubitus ulcers.

Projectile vomiting—sudden forceful vomiting.

Prone—lying face down.

Prostatectomy—removal of the prostate gland in the male.

Psychiatrist—a specialist in the treatment of diseases of the mind.

Puberty—the period when the reproductive organs become capable of functioning.

Pulse—the throbbing of arteries reflecting the heart beat.

Puncture wound—a small, deep opening in the skin caused by a piercing instrument or weapon.

Range of motion—the range of movement possible for any given joint.

Rash—a skin eruption.

Rectum—the last eight to ten inches of the large intestines where feces are stored.

Regurgitation—the spitting up of undigested food.

Rehabilitation—restoring to optimal health.

Respiration—the act of breathing.

Roughage—foods rich in cellulose and residue.

Saliva—the secretions of the glands of the mouth intended to moisten and aid in swallowing food.

Salmonella—a type of bacteria capable of causing acute intestinal upset, found in food and water.

Sebaceous glands—glands in the skin which secrete oil.

Sedative—a medication which calms excitement.

Shock—an upset caused by inadequate blood circulation resulting in pallor; rapid, weak pulse; and pale, clammy skin.

Sordes—filth and crusts that accumulate on the lips and in the mouth of seriously ill or unconscious patients especially during a high fever.

Spasm—a sudden muscular contraction.

Sputum—material from the throat and mouth discharged by spitting.

Sternum—flat, narrow bone to which the ribs are connected in front.

Stool—feces, a bowel movement.

Stridor—harsh, vibrating respirations.

Stupor—a partly conscious but lethargic state.

Supine—lying face up.

Suppurate—to form pus.

Susceptible—a person who lacks immunity and is apt to contract a disease if exposed.

Symptom—an evidence of disease.

Theraputic—related to the treatment of disease.

Thermal burns—burns caused by heat.

Trauma—a wound or injury. In psychiatry a deep emotional shock leaving a lasting impression.

Void—to empty the contents of the bladder.

Volatile—vaporizes readily.

Vomitus—vomited matter.

Wound—an injury to the body in which tissue is damaged. An open wound is a break in the skin or mucous membrane.

INDEX

A

health, 4
Avulsion, first aid for the, 127-28

B

Back rub, 61-62
Backrests, improvised, for the sick room, 149-51
Bargaining, as a stage of terminal illness, 102
Basic four food groups, and nutrition, 4-5
Bath, for the bedfast patient, procedure for, 58-61
Bath blanket, and the bath, 59
Bath mitt, making the, 59
Bathroom, safety hazards in the, 107
Bed
    methods of elevating, 21, 147-48
    requirements of the, in the sick room, 21
    single, and body mechanics, 46
    special improvised equipment for, in the sick room, 147-49
Bed bag, construction of the, for the sick room, 154-55
Bed making, procedure for, for the bedfast patient, 62-67
Bed table, 52
Bedpan
    improvisation of the, 153
    use of, 55-56
    warming of, 55
    washing of, 56
Bedside equipment, for bedfast patient, 21-22, 68
Bedsores, 47, 61, 63, 92
Behavior, and illness, 36
Black eye, cause of, 136
Blanket, protection of the, 66
Bleaches, poisoning by, 105
Bleeding

care of, 126-28
control of, 114
first aid for, 128
from nose, ear, or mouth, and brain injury, 135-36
selecting cloth used to stop, 117
and shock, 124
Blood type, and family health records, 12
Body elimination, unusual, and illness, 35
Body mechanics, 45-48
Bone, injuries to, first aid for, 134-36
Bones, danger of breakage of, in aged, 90
Book rack, construction of the, for the sick room, 155
Brain, symptoms of injury to, 135-36
Brain Tumors, and behavior change, 36
Bread, daily requirements of, 5
Bread-cereal group, and the full liquid diet, 72
Bruises, first aid for, 127
Burning, rescue from, 142
Burns
    first aid for, 132-34
    and shock, 124, 133
    three degrees of, 132-33
    treatment of, 132-33

C

Caffeine, and aspirin, 80
Cancer
    prevention or detection of, 2
    seven danger signals of, 36-37
    and smoking, 3
Carbon monoxide, as an inhaled poison, 130
Carbon monoxide poisoning,

and respiratory failure, 120
Cardiac massage, 114
Cardiopulmonary resuscitation,
    use of, 124
Cardiovascular changes, and
    aging, 87
Castor oil, as a laxative, 81
Cataracts, 89
Cathartics, 81
Cereal, daily requirements of, 5
Charcoal, medicinal activated, as
    an antidote, 130
Chemical burns, first aid for,
    133
Chemicals, as a cause of burns,
    132
Chicken pox, 10
Children
    aspirin dosage for, 79-80
    and burns, 132
    care for sick, 25-28
    and cleaning materials,
        106
    and clear liquid diet, 72
    and constipation, 57
    and convulsions, 118
    dangers to, in the home,
        105
    and detergents, 106
    diversions for sick, 27-28
    giving medicine to, 83-84
    and hospitalization, 27
    and insecticides, 106
    and medicine, 106
    mouth-to-mouth resuscita-
        tion for, 122-24
    observation of illness in, 33
    and pain, 36
    and pesticides, 106
    and poisoning, 129
    sick, and food, 75
    temperature taking and
        fever in, 41
    transportation of, with
        injuries, 140-41
Chlorine, compounds from, as
    an inhaled poison, 130

Choking, and poisoning, 129
Circulation
    and cyanosis, 34
    importance of good, for
        the patient, 47
Cirrhosis of the liver, and
    jaundice, 34
Cloth, sterilization of, for dress-
    ings, 117
Clothing, appropriate, for the
    aged, 96-97
Coffee, and harmful stimulants, 3
Colas, and harmful stimulants, 3
Cold, as a treatment, 86, 127,
    134
Cold remedies, value of, 81-82
Comfort, and home nursing, 19
Commode chair, 56, 153
Confinement in bed, problems
    of, for aged, 92
Conjunctivitis, 11, 35
Constipation
    and the bedfast patient,
        56-57
    and laxatives, 80
    as a symptom, 35
Contractures, 46
Convalescence, of the sick child,
    27-28
Convulsions
    and brain injury, 136
    causes of, 118
    first aid for, 118
    and poisoning, 129
Cooper, Dr. Kenneth, and
    aerobics, 2
Croup, and respiratory failure,
    120
Cut, first aid for the, 127
Cyanosis
    and illness, 34
    and respiratory failure, 120

D

Death
    acceptance of one's own,

E

of, 137
Ears, foreign objects in, first aid
  for, 137
Economy, and home nursing, 20
Eczema, 34
Ego, illness and the, 28-29
Electrocution
  rescue from, 142
  and respiratory failure,
    120
Emergency, preparedness for,
  13-17
Emesis basin, and mouth care,
  58
Emphysema
  and cyanosis, 34
  and smoking, 3
Enema, and constipation, 57
Epilepsy, and convulsions, 118
Exercise
  and the aged, 95
  importance of, 1
Eyes
  and chemical burns, 131
  foreign objects in, first aid
    for, 136-37
  inflammation of, 35
  sign of illness in, 34-35
  sunburn of, 136
  unequal size of pupils of,
    and brain injury, 136

F

Face, fractures of, first aid for,
  138
Fainting
  causes of, 118
  recovery from, 118
Falls, prevention of, 106
Family, protection of, from
  communicable diseases, 12
Feet, problems with, in aged,
  90-91
Fever
  and convulsions, 118
  and pulse, 43

reduction of, 41
and respiration, 43
and the sick child, 27
First aid, 113-43
  definition of, 113
  improvised equipment for,
    117
  legal implications of,
    114-15
  principles of, after an
    accident, 113-14
First-aid kit, 115-17
First-degree burns, first aid for,
  132
Food, storage of, for emergency
  use, 14-15
Food poisoning, and abdominal
  pain, 119
Fractures, first aid for, 134-35
Frostbite, first aid for, 144
Fruit, daily requirements of, 5

G

Gall bladder, diseases of the, and
  jaundice, 34
Gallstones, and abdominal pain,
  119
Gas, as an inhaled poison, 130
German Measles, 8, 10
Glaucoma, 89
Good Samaritan laws, and first
  aid, 115
Gums, deterioration of, in aged,
  90

H

Hair
  care of, of patient, 67-68
  changes in, of aged, 91
Handwashing, and the spread of
  infection, 22, 24
Head injury, and convulsions,
  118
Headache, and brain injury, 134
Health, definition of, 1

Infection
    prevention of spread of,
        22-25
    and shock, 125
Infectious Hepatitis, 10
Influenza, 9
Insect poisoning, 131
Insecticides
    care of, 106
    poisoning by, 105
Insomnia, and the depressed
    patient, 29
Insulin, and the diabetic, 119
Ipecac, syrup of, to induce
    vomiting, 130

J

Jaw, fractures of, first aid for,
    138
Jaundice, 34
Joints, injuries to the, first aid
    for, 134-36

K

Kerosene, poisoning by, 105
Kidney stones, and abdominal
    pain, 119
Kitchen, safety hazards in the,
    107

L

Laceration, first aid for the, 127
Laxatives
    and constipation, 57
    dependence on, 3
    four main types of, 80-81
    lubricant, 80-81
    use of, 80
Leisure time, use of, by aged, 99
Leukemia, and behavior change,
    36
Light, in the sick room, 21

Listlessness, and the depressed
    patient, 29
Liver, cancer of the, and jaun-
    dice, 34
Lung disease, prevention or de-
    tection of, 2

M

Malaise, and illness, 36
Marine life poisoning, 131
Mattress
    height of, and body
        mechanics, 46
    requirements of the, in the
        sick room, 21
Meals, rules for preparation of,
    73-74
Measles, 9, 10
Meat, daily requirements of, 5
Meat group, and the full liquid
    diet, 72
Medical checkups
    during menopause, 95
    importance of regular, 2
Medical record, personal, 6-7
Medications
    disposal of old, 85
    in first-aid kit, 117
    liquid, and babies, 84
Medicines
    and accident victims, 114
    and children, 83-84, 106
    common, used in the
        home, 79-82
    expiration date of, 84
    keeping prescription,
        84-85
    principles of giving, in the
        home, 82-84
    rules for care of, in the
        home, 84
    storage of, 106
Memory, weakening of, in aged,
    98-99
Meningitis, 10
    and convulsions, 118

Redness, of skin, and illness, 34
Regression, and illness, 28
Relaxation, importance of, 1
Religion, and the seriously ill, 30
Rescue
    of accident victim, 138-42
    methods of, 139-42
    situations requiring im-
        mediate, 139
Respiration
    counting of, 42-43
    and fever, 43
    as a sign of shock, 123
    as a vital sign, 35
Respiratory failure
    causes of, 120
    signs of, 120
    first aid for, 119-24
Respiratory system, and aging,
    88
Rest, importance of, 1
Resuscitation
    cardiopulmonary, use of,
        124
    mouth-to-mouth, 120-24
Rheumatic fever, and sore
    throat, 38
Ringworm of the scalp, 11
Rubella. See German Measles
Rubeola. See Measles

S

Safety
    and home nursing, 19
    rules for, in the home,
        105-11
Salmonellosis, 11
Scabies, 11
Scalp wounds, first aid for, 135
Second-degree burns, first aid
    for, 132
Sedatives, dependence on, 3
Senses, and aging, 88-89
Sex, and aging, 94-95
Sheet
    pulling the, tight, 65

    squaring the corner of the,
        63-64
Sheet blanket, and the bath, 59
Shock
    and accident victims, 114
    and burns, 131
    causes of, 124-25
    emergency protection
        from, 125-26
    signs of, 125
Sick room
    daily schedule of activities
        in, 69-70
    neatness of, and home
        nursing, 20
    setting up the, 20-22
Sight, lessening of sense of, in
    aged, 89
Signs, versus symptoms, 33
Skin
    changes in, of aged, 91
    changes in color of, and
        illness, 34
    color of, as a sign of
        shock, 125
Skin temperature, and illness, 34
Skull fracture, 135
Sleep, and the aged, 95
Sleepiness, and poisoning, 129
Smallpox, 9
Smell, lessening of sense of, in
    aged, 88
Smoking, and cancer and em-
    physema, 3
Snakebite, first aid for, 130-31
Snowburn, first aid for, 144-45
Sordes, prevention of, 58
Speech, disturbances of, and
    brain injury, 136
Splinting, methods of, 135
Sponge bath, and fever, 41
Sprain, treatment for, 134
Sterile dressings, preparation of,
    116
Strangulation, and respiratory
    failure, 120
Strep Throat, 11
Stroke, 118

Stroke patient, helping the, to walk, 54
Suffocation, rescue from, 142
Suicide, and the depressed patient, 29
Sunburn, first aid for, 133
Sunstroke, first aid for, 143
Suppository, and constipation, 57
Symptoms, versus signs, 33

T

Taste, lessening of sense of, in aged, 88
Tea, and harmful stimulants, 3
Teeth, deterioration of, in aged, 89-90
Temperature
    axillary, 41
    drop in body, and shock, 125
    maintaining normal, in accident victims, 114
    recording of, 41, 42
    rectal, 41
    in the sick room, 21
    of the skin, and illness, 34
    taking of, 38-42
    as a vital sign, 35
Terminal illness, stages of, 101-4
Tetanus, 8
Thermometer
    breaking of, in patient's mouth, 42
    clinical, parts of, 38-40
    clinical, use of, 40-41
    in first-aid kit, 116
    rectal, and axillary temperature, 41
    rectal, use of, 41
Third-degree burns, first aid for, 133
Thirst, as a sign of shock, 125
Throat
    inspection of, 37-38
    signs of illness in, 35

    swollen, as a sign of illness, 38
Toe space, bedding pleated for, 66
Tongue depressor, 38
Tonsils, 37
Tooth decay, prevention of, 3
Touch, lessening of sense of, in aged, 88
Tourniquet, use of, 128
Tranquilizers, dependence on, 3
Transportation, of accident victim, 138-42
Typhoid fever, 9

U

Ulcers
    and abdominal pain, 119
    and mental health, 4
Unconsciousness
    and brain injury, 136
    and poisoning, 129
    possible causes of, 118-19
Urinal
    for the bedfast male, 55
    improvisations of the, 152-53
Urination, frequency of or burning upon, as a symptom, 35

V

Vegetables, daily requirements of, 5
Vegetables and fruit group, and the full liquid diet, 72
Vital signs, 35
    recording of, 43
Vitamin supplements, value of, 82
Vocal cords, swelling of, and respiratory failure, 120
Volatile liquids, vapors from, as an inhaled poison, 130
Vomiting

and brain injury, 135
and clear liquid diet, 71
ipecac syrup to induce, in
first-aid kit, 117
and poisoning, 129
and poisons, 129-30
and shock, 124
and the sick child, 27
as a sign of shock, 125
as a symptom, 35

W

Waste disposal
avoidance of inadequate, 3
and the spread of infec-
tion, 22
Waste elimination
and the bedfast patient,
55-57
improvised equipment for,
in the sick room,
152-53
problems of, of aged,
91-92

Water
methods of disinfecting,
16
storage of, for emergency
use, 13
Weakness, and mental health, 4
Weight, and family health
records, 12
Wheelchair, use of, 54
Whooping cough, 8, 11
Withdrawal, and the depressed
patient, 29
Worthlessness, feelings of, and
the depressed patient, 29
Wounds
care of, 126-28
cleansing of, 128
closed, 127
open, 126-27
open, types of, 127-28

X

X-rays, and family health
records, 12

ABOUT THE AUTHOR

Alice M. Schmidt, R.N., is well qualified to be the author of a home nursing text. Mother of six children, three girls and three boys, she has combined a career in nursing and teaching with caring for her husband and her children—including childhood diseases, lacerations, and other ailments. Not only has she cared for her own family, she has frequently been in demand in her neighborhood when physical ailments have struck the homes of her friends.

Although she had not planned to become a nurse and did so "quite by accident" in searching for a suitable major during her college days, she has found it a deeply rewarding career, contributing toward the success of her marriage and the care of her family. Asked how she came to write *The Homemaker's Guide to Home Nursing,* she replied that she felt the majority of homemakers need such a handbook:

In recent years as my teaching responsibilities have moved away from working with majors in nursing to non-nursing students, I have become increasingly aware of the insecurity women feel in dealing with illness in the home. It is to help these homemakers that I have written this book, hoping it will serve as a resource when hubby thinks he's coming down with the flu or when Junior falls out of a tree. It does not have all the answers, but hopefully it has many of them.

Mrs. Schmidt is an assistant professor in the College of Nursing at Brigham Young University, a Red Cross instructor-trainer in home nursing, and a lecturer at workshops on home nursing for Continuing Education in the West. She is also a member of the Red Cross, the Utah Nurses Association, and the National League of Nurses. For about fifteen years, intermittently, from 1954 to 1970, she acquired practical experience as a nurse in hospitals. A doctoral candidate at BYU in Educational Administration, she has written lessons on home nursing for the women's organization of The Church of Jesus Christ of Latter-day Saints for the last four years. This book draws liberally from those lessons and from the materials she has used in her teaching career.